THE HOLISTIC PARASITE DETOX

RESTORING HEALTH NATURALLY FROM THE INSIDE OUT

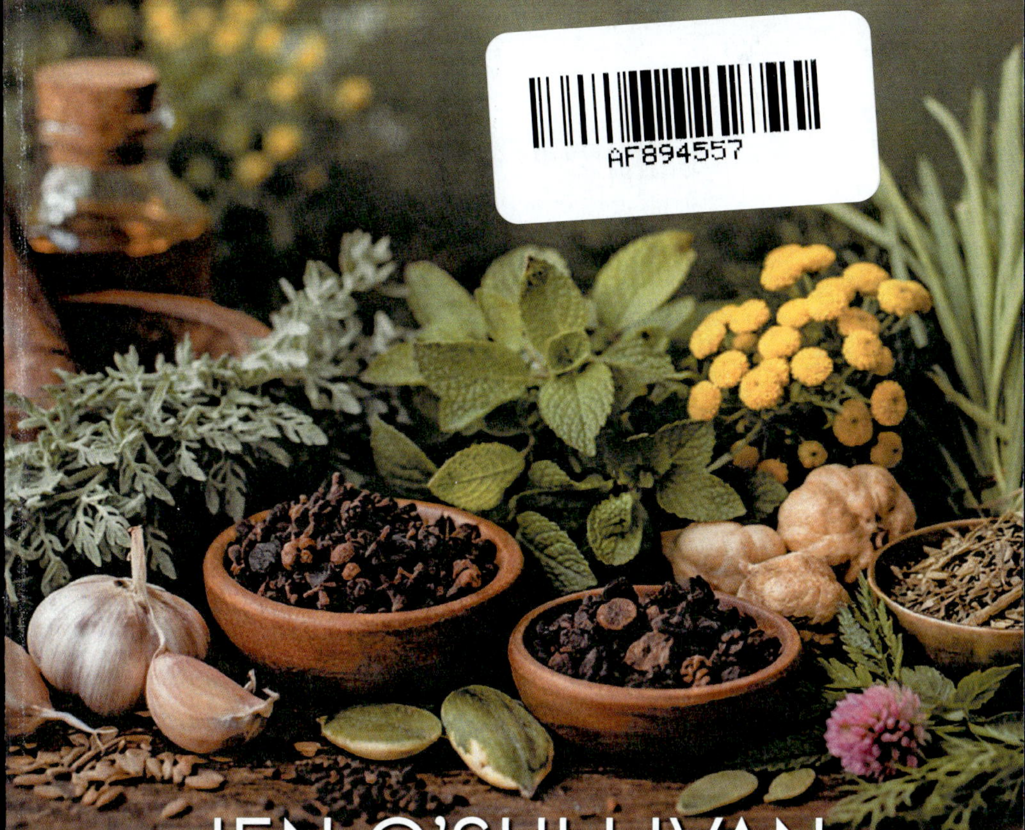

JEN O'SULLIVAN

BOARD CERTIFIED NATUROPATHIC PRACTITIONER
& CERTIFIED MASTER HERBALIST

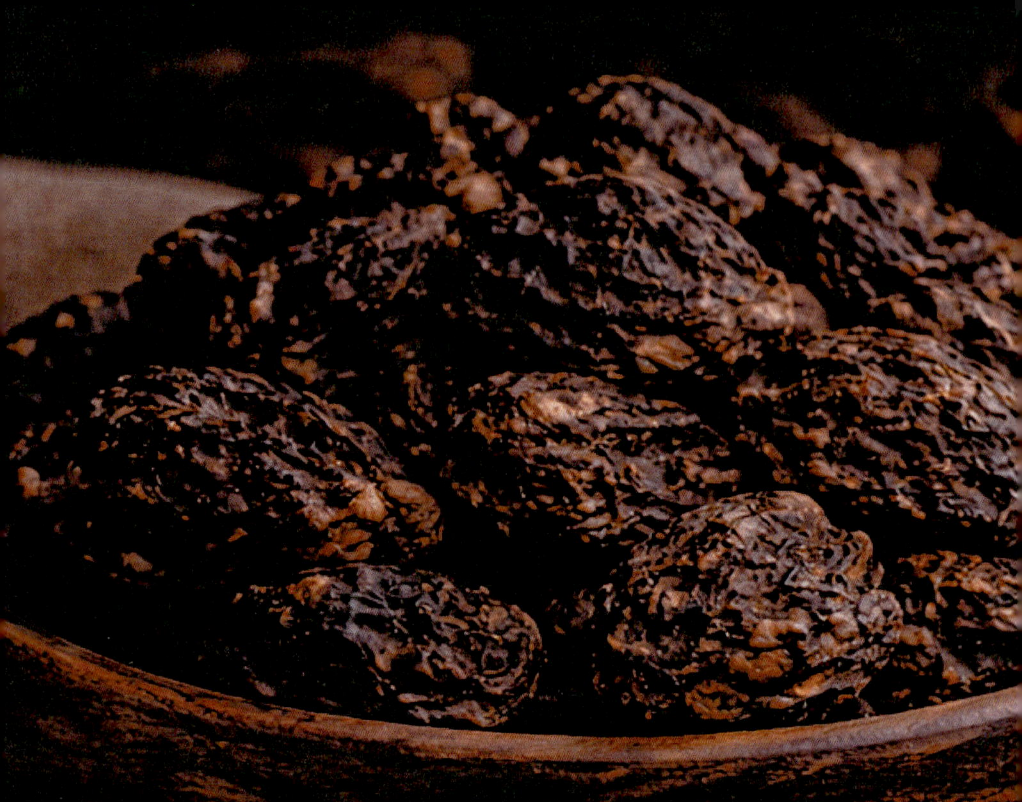

THE HOLISTIC PARASITE DETOX

Cover design by Jen O'Sullivan

Technical Editor: Sandra Kozij
General and Copy Editors: Sandra Kozij, Diane Finefrock, Christine Rodriguez, Diane Fischer, and Kathy Schwanke

Published March 2026
www.JenOSullivan.com

ISBN: 978-1-969090-02-8

CANYON HOUSE
PUBLISHING

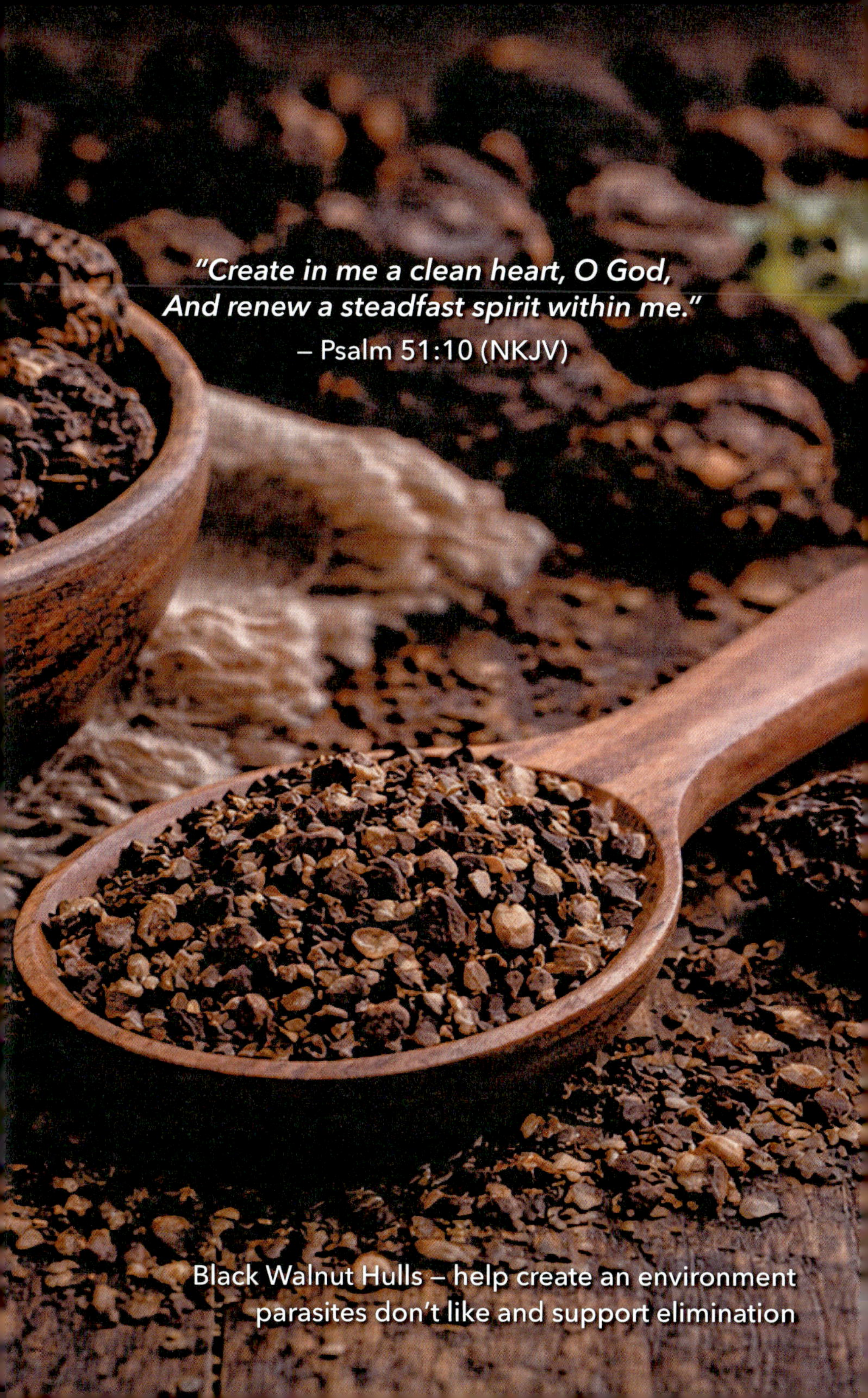

"Create in me a clean heart, O God,
And renew a steadfast spirit within me."
– Psalm 51:10 (NKJV)

Black Walnut Hulls – help create an environment parasites don't like and support elimination

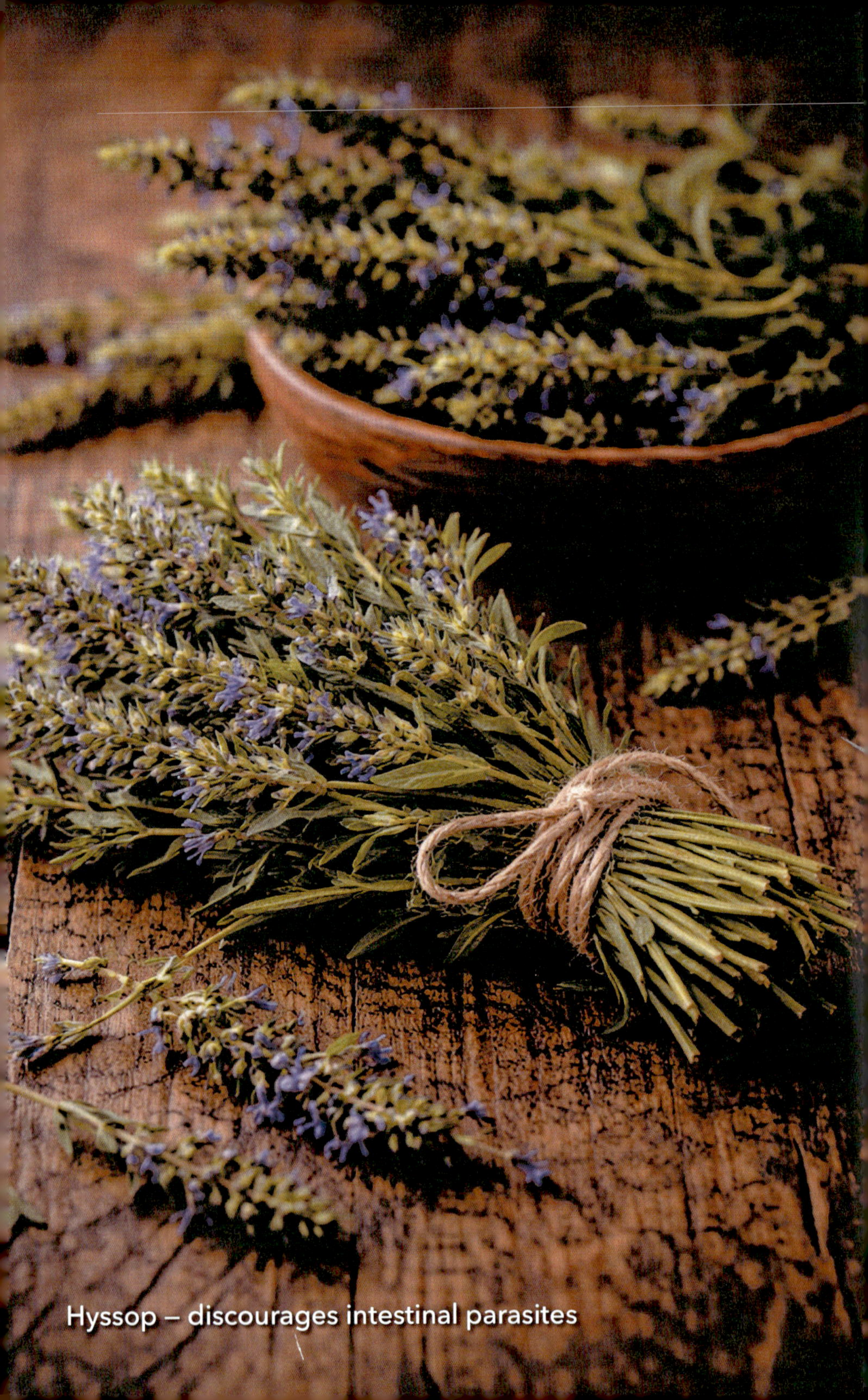

Hyssop – discourages intestinal parasites

CONTENTS

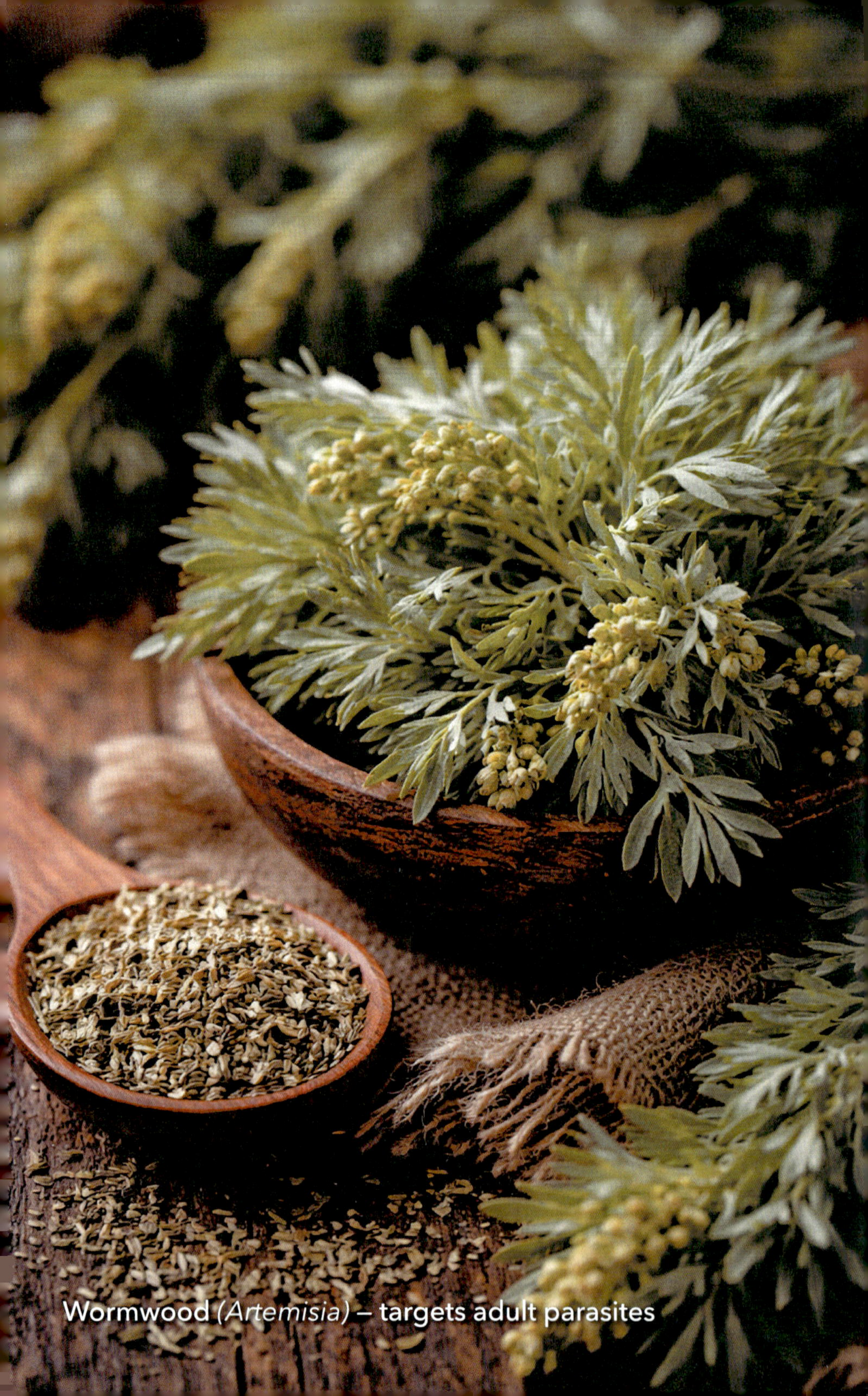

Wormwood *(Artemisia)* – targets adult parasites

INTRODUCTION

PARASITES – THE HIDDEN HEALTH BURDEN

Drain the swamp. Eliminate the invaders. Kill the parasites. Maybe this seems extreme, but consider this: have you been quietly suffering from unexplainable mood swings, fatigue that comes out of nowhere, bloating, inflammation, brain fog, skin issues, sleep disturbances, immune response decline, unexplained food sensitivities? The symptom list can be overwhelming, and these are just a few common symptoms. Once you drain the swamp, aka perform a parasite detox, you may be shocked to feel many of your unexplained symptoms lift or clear entirely.

Many people spend years chasing symptoms without ever asking a deeper question. What is driving this pattern? It is easy to label issues as hormonal, stress-related, or simply part of aging. Those factors matter, yet they often sit on top of something else. When the root is overlooked, the cycle continues. You manage, cope, adjust, and push through. Meanwhile, the underlying burden remains untouched.

That is what makes parasites so deceptive. They rarely demand attention in obvious ways. They quietly take, slowly influence, and subtly interfere. Over time, the body adapts to their presence. What once felt abnormal begins to feel familiar. Energy dips become routine. Digestive discomfort becomes expected. Mental fog becomes something you work around instead of question.

Parasites are usually associated with remote regions, unsafe water, or extreme poverty. Most people do not picture them as part of everyday modern life. Yet they remain one of the most overlooked contributors of chronic imbalance in developed nations. They move quietly, often unnoticed, like tenants who never signed a lease but keep helping themselves to the pantry.

By definition, a parasite survives by feeding on a host. It draws nourishment without contributing to the system that sustains it. Inside the human body, this can mean competition for nutrients, irritation of tissues, increased toxic load, and disruption of normal immune communication. Some provoke inflammation. Others release metabolic waste. Many persist without obvious symptoms, blending into the background of daily function.

Another layer to consider is how they influence behavior and signaling. Cravings, especially for sugar and refined carbohydrates, can become stronger and harder to manage. Appetite can feel inconsistent. Mood can shift without a clear reason. These patterns are not always about willpower. They can reflect deeper biological interference that pulls the body out of alignment.

The assumption that parasites exist only in distant places no longer fits modern conditions. International travel, imported foods, shared water systems, and large-scale agriculture have dissolved old geographic boundaries. Exposure has become ordinary rather than exceptional.

Undercooked meat, unwashed produce, contaminated water, contact with animals, walking barefoot on soil, and improperly cleaned food surfaces all provide entry points. Parasites do not require extreme environments. They require opportunity, which modern living supplies.

Food now travels thousands of miles before reaching the plate. Produce passes through countless hands. Animals are raised in dense populations. Water is filtered and reused through massive municipal systems. At the same time, stress, processed foods, medications, and disrupted sleep patterns weaken gut barriers and immune signaling.

The terrain has shifted, defenses are often weakened, and as a result, unwanted exposures occur more easily than most people realize.

Parasites do not always announce themselves with dramatic symptoms. Many behave more like static in the body's communication systems. Fatigue that never fully resolves. Cravings that feel out of proportion. Skin eruptions that migrate. Digestive discomfort without a clear pattern. Immune systems that remain stuck in a low-grade state of alarm.

A helpful image is stagnant water. Mosquitoes do not create the swamp. They take advantage of it. The real issue is not the insect but the conditions that allow it to multiply. This is why detoxification must be approached with intention.

There is also a timing component that often gets ignored. The body has rhythms. Detox pathways follow order. Elimination depends on readiness. When that order is respected, the process is smoother and more effective. When it is rushed, the body pushes back. What feels like resistance is often protection.

The body is an ecosystem, so a mindful approach to removing parasites is key. Harsh or rapid cleansing can overload the liver, strain the kidneys, disturb mineral balance, and provoke stress responses. When parasites die too quickly, stored toxins and metabolic waste enter circulation. Without proper elimination support, this creates congestion rather than resolution. What many call a "detox reaction" is often a traffic jam in the body's drainage systems.

Draining the swamp requires channels. Killing organisms without supporting elimination simply spreads the debris.

A structured approach respects physiology. It prepares detox pathways. It strengthens gut integrity. It supports immune coordination. It reduces reinfection risk. Only then does it address unwanted organisms.

This book exists to increase an understanding of parasites, explain systems, and give grounded guidance. It does not replace medical care. It serves as education and framework. Biology is too complex for shortcuts or universal solutions.

Within these pages, you will learn how parasites enter the body, how they persist, and how the body is designed to remove them when supported appropriately. The focus will be on stewardship, order, and preparation.

What you will learn:

- how exposure occurs
- how parasites affect digestion, immunity, and detoxification
- why timing and pacing matter
- how to support elimination pathways
- how to strengthen the internal terrain

What you will not learn:

- disease diagnosis
- one-size-fits-all prescriptions
- aggressive cleansing methods
- miracle claims
- reckless protocols

Education sharpens discernment, and discernment protects health. Parasites thrive in darkness, but light reveals what needs to be addressed and what needs to be strengthened. Let's dig in!

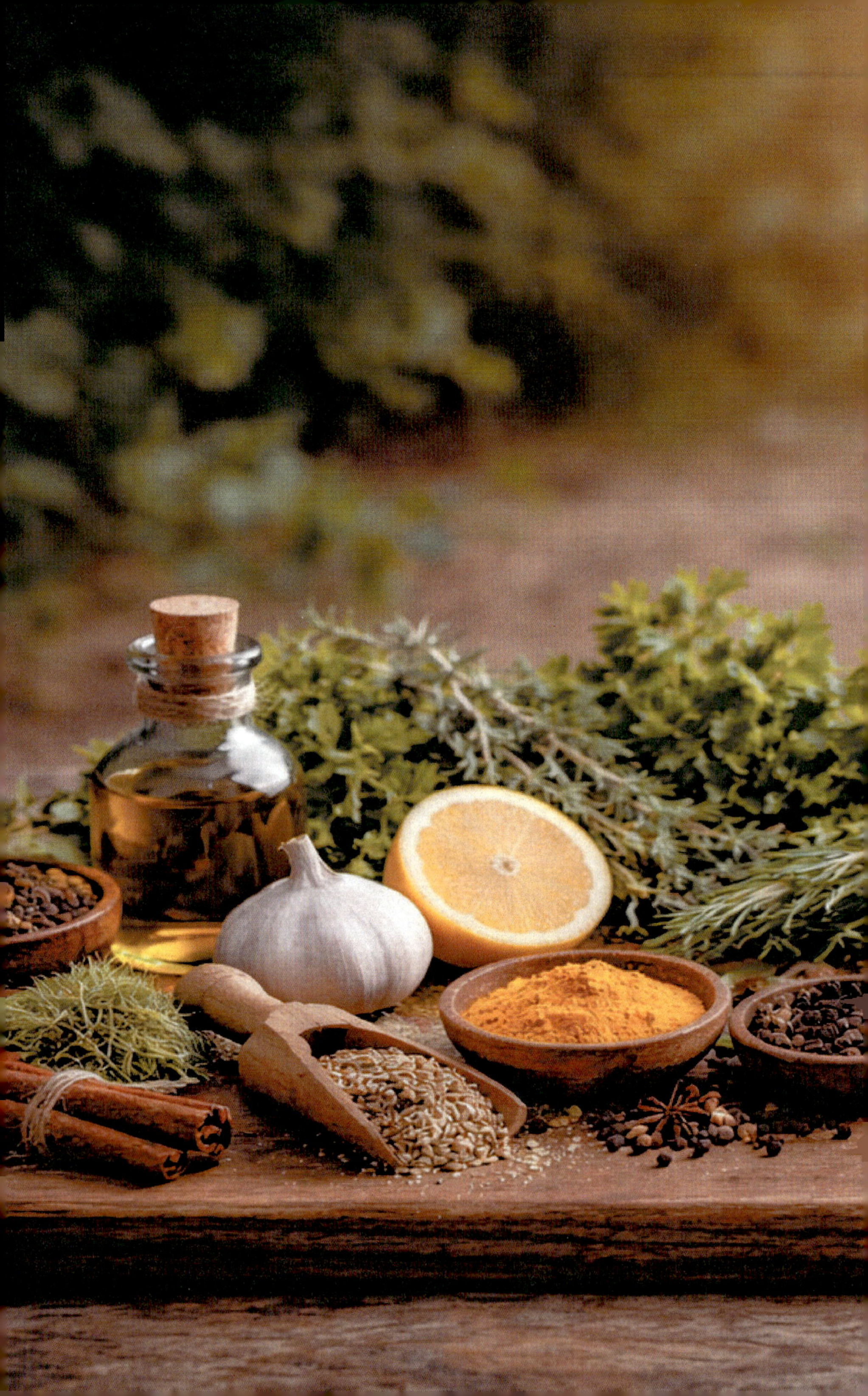

PART ONE

PARASITE BASICS

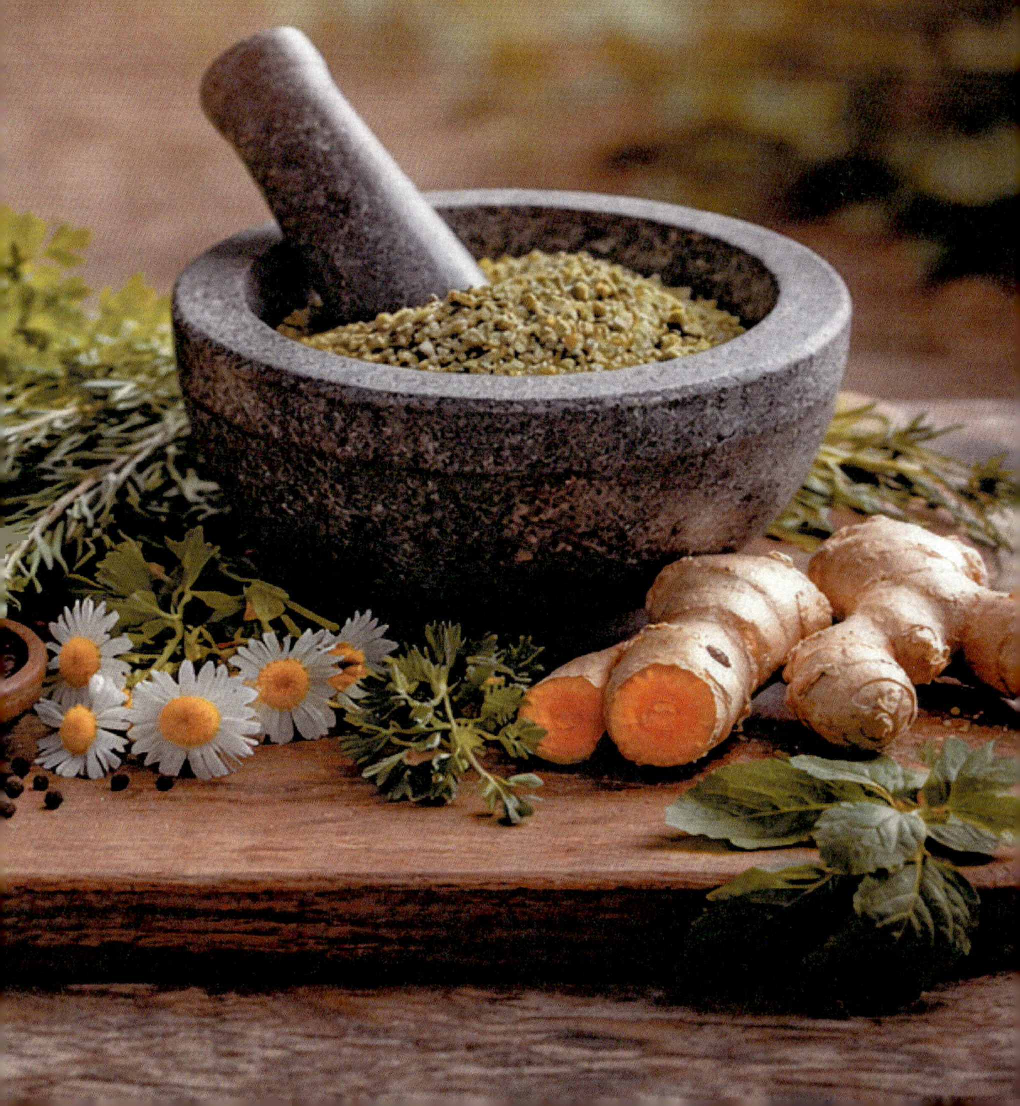

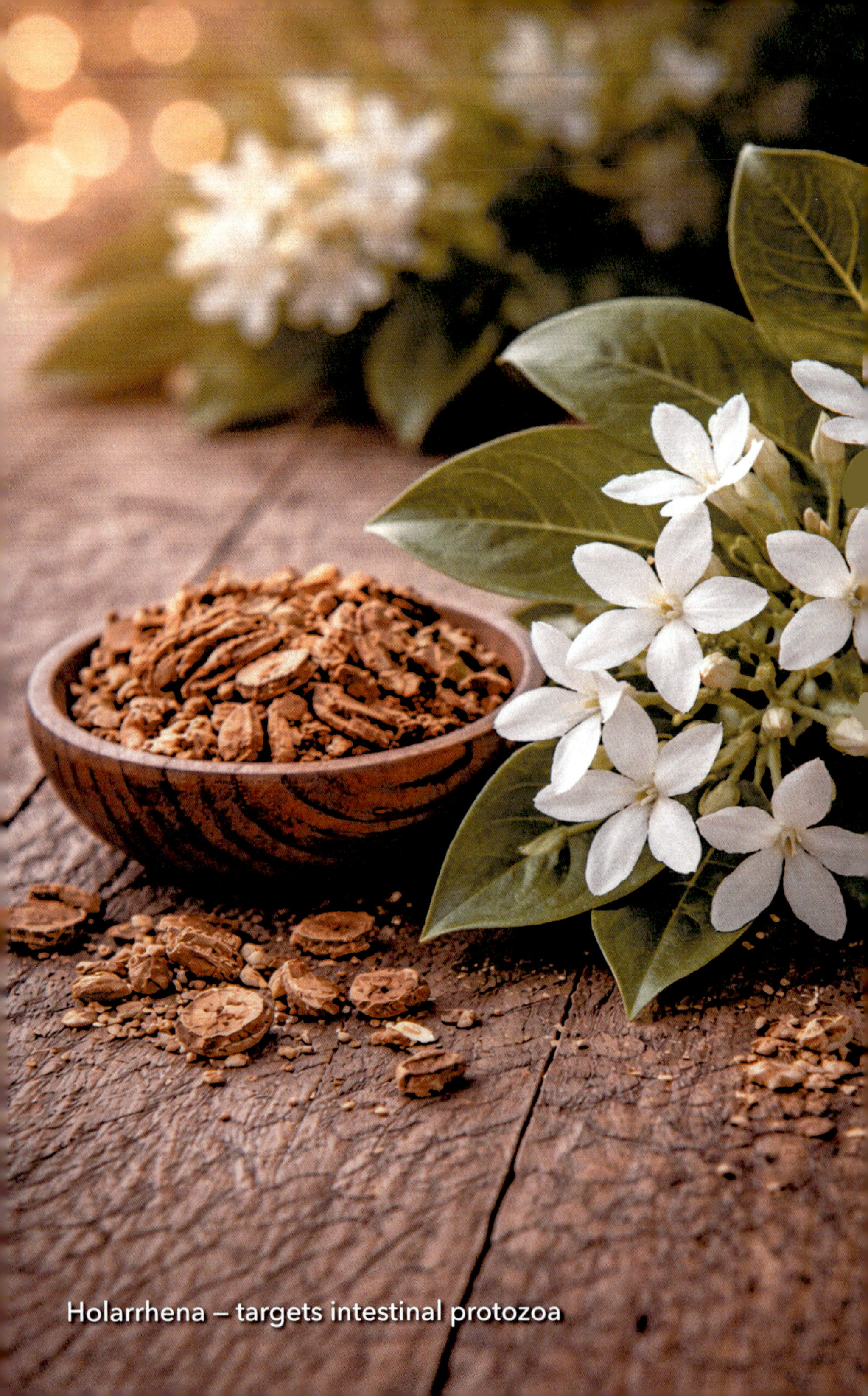

Holarrhena – targets intestinal protozoa

CHAPTER 1
UNDERSTANDING PARASITES

Parasites have shared the earth with all living forms, including humans, since the beginning of time. They are not a modern problem, nor are they limited to "third-world" countries or unsanitary living conditions. Parasites exist everywhere there is life. They exist in soil, water, animals, and humans. The real issue is not whether parasites exist, but whether the body is able to keep them in check.

A parasite is an organism that lives in or on another organism and depends on it for survival. Unlike beneficial bacteria that work with the body, parasites live at the host's expense. They consume nutrients, release metabolic waste, and disrupt normal biological processes. Some are large enough to see with the naked eye, while others are so small they require a microscope to detect.

WHAT PARASITES ARE

Parasites generally fall into three broad categories: worms, protozoa, and microscopic parasites.

Worm parasites, also called helminths, include roundworms, tapeworms, hookworms, and flukes. These organisms can live in the intestines, liver, lungs, blood, and even muscle tissue. Some grow several feet long and can survive inside the human body for years if conditions allow.

Protozoa are single-celled organisms that behave very differently from worms. They multiply rapidly and can invade tissues, blood, and organs. Common protozoan parasites include organisms that affect the digestive tract and those that travel through the bloodstream. Because of their small size and rapid reproduction, protozoa can cause widespread symptoms in a short period of time.

Microscopic parasites include organisms such as certain fungi-like microbes and blood-borne parasites. These are often overlooked because they do not resemble what people traditionally imagine when they think of a parasite. Yet they can interfere with immune signaling, oxygen delivery, and nutrient absorption just as effectively as larger organisms.

Together, these organisms form a hidden biological ecosystem within the human body when conditions permit their survival.

HOW PARASITES SURVIVE INSIDE THE HUMAN BODY

Parasites are biologically designed to survive hostile environments. The human body, with its warmth, moisture, and steady food supply, is an ideal habitat.

Many parasites survive by evading immune detection. Some change their surface proteins so the immune system does not recognize them as invaders. Others hide inside tissues or cells, where they are shielded from immune attack. Certain species can even suppress immune responses in their surrounding environment, creating a localized zone where they can live undisturbed.

Parasites feed on glucose, iron, amino acids, and vitamins taken in through the diet. This means the host may be consuming adequate nutrition yet still experiencing deficiencies because nutrients are being diverted. Over time, this can weaken tissues, impair detoxification pathways, and disrupt hormone production.

Some parasites also release chemicals that affect digestion and gut motility. This helps them remain attached to intestinal walls and slows their removal. Their waste products, known as metabolic byproducts, can trigger inflammation and place additional stress on the liver and immune system. Parasites thrive in a weakened or overburdened body.

COMMON MYTHS VS. BIOLOGICAL REALITY

One of the most common myths is that parasites only infect people who travel internationally or live in unsanitary conditions. In reality, parasites are contracted through food, water, soil, pets, insect bites, and even person-to-person contact. Undercooked meat, unwashed produce, contaminated water, and exposure to animals are all common transmission routes.

Another myth is that parasites always cause dramatic symptoms. Many people assume that unless they see worms in stool or experience extreme digestive distress, parasites cannot be present. Biologically, this is inaccurate. Parasites often aim to remain undetected so they can survive longer. Subtle symptoms such as fatigue, nutrient deficiencies, skin issues, and mood changes are more common than obvious signs.

There is also a belief that parasites can only live in the intestines. In reality, parasites have been found in the liver, lungs, brain, muscles, and bloodstream. Their location in the body influences which symptoms appear, making detection more complex than a simple stool test.

The idea that stomach acid or cooking foods to a specific temperature prevents parasites entirely is another oversimplification. While stomach acid and cooking foods thoroughly are important defenses, many parasites survive harsh conditions by forming protective cysts or eggs that resist digestion and hatch later in the intestines. Biological reality is far more adaptive and resilient than popular assumptions.

WHY SYMPTOMS VARY SO WIDELY

One of the greatest challenges in identifying parasitic burden is that symptoms differ dramatically from person to person. Two individuals can host similar organisms and experience completely different outcomes.

This variation depends on several factors. Immune function plays a major role. A strong, well-regulated immune system may suppress parasite activity, keeping symptoms mild or nonexistent. A weakened immune system may allow rapid growth and migration, leading to more severe manifestations.

Nutritional status also matters. A body already low in minerals, protein, or antioxidants is more vulnerable to damage from parasitic waste and nutrient theft. Stress levels, sleep quality, toxin exposure, and gut health further influence how the body responds.

Location matters as well. Parasites in the intestines may cause bloating, diarrhea, or constipation. Parasites in the bloodstream may contribute to fatigue, brain fog, or temperature dysregulation. Parasites affecting tissues or organs may present as pain, inflammation, or unexplained immune reactions.

Some people experience skin symptoms such as rashes or itching. Others experience anxiety, insomnia, or irritability. Still others struggle with weight changes, cravings, or chronic inflammation. These differences do not mean parasites are absent. They reflect how uniquely each body adapts to biological stress.

A BROADER PERSPECTIVE

Understanding parasites requires a shift in perspective. They flourish when terrain allows it. A body burdened by toxins, poor digestion, chronic stress, and weakened detox pathways creates an environment where parasites can thrive. Recognizing parasites as part of a broader imbalance opens the door to meaningful restoration. Addressing terrain, detoxification, immune support, and microbial balance becomes just as important as removing the organisms themselves. Parasites reveal what the body can no longer manage quietly.

In the chapters ahead, you will explore how parasites enter the body, the symptoms they may cause, and why cleansing must be done thoughtfully rather than aggressively. Understanding their biology is the first step toward reclaiming internal balance and restoring the body's natural capacity to defend itself. Before parasites can be removed, they must be understood.

KEY TERMS FROM THIS SECTION

- **Parasite** – an organism that lives at another organism's expense
- **Host** – the organism (human) that the parasite lives in or on
- **Helminths** – a category of parasitic worms
- **Protozoa** – single-celled parasitic organisms
- **Microscopic parasites** – extremely small parasites
- **Metabolic waste/byproducts** – produced by parasites
- **Immune detection** – the immune system's ability to recognize threats
- **Surface proteins** – immune system "labels" to recognize organisms
- **Immune suppression** – the reduction of immune response
- **Glucose** – a form of sugar used for energy
- **Amino acids** – building blocks of protein
- **Detoxification pathways** – systems in the body (especially liver and gut) that remove toxins
- **Pathways** – the routes the body uses to carry out important jobs
- **Gut motility** – the movement of food/waste through digestion
- **Inflammation** – the body's response to injury or irritation
- **Transmission routes** – ways parasites enter the body
- **Cysts** – protective shells some parasites form to survive
- **Parasitic burden** – the total load of parasites in the body
- **Manifestations** – how symptoms show up in the body
- **Terrain** – the environment of the body, both good and bad
- **Microbial balance** – the balance of bacteria, fungi, and other microorganisms in the body
- **Biological ecosystem** – the interacting organisms living in the body
- **Adaptive** – able to change or survive under different conditions
- **Resilient** – able to withstand stress or damage
- **Dysregulation** – loss of normal control or balance (immune function)

ORGANS, PARASITES, & SYMPTOMS

This section organizes common human parasites by the primary organ or body system they most often affect, beginning with the most commonly involved areas and progressing to the least common. For each body system, the most frequently encountered parasites are listed along with their typical sources of exposure and the symptoms they most commonly produce.

INTESTINES (most common site)

- **Ascaris (roundworms)**
  Obtained Through: contaminated food, water, soil
  Common Symptoms: abdominal pain, bloating, diarrhea, malnutrition
- **Hookworms**
  Obtained Through: bare feet on contaminated soil
  Common Symptoms: anemia, fatigue, itchy feet, diarrhea
- **Strongyloides**
  Obtained Through: skin contact with contaminated soil
  Common Symptoms: diarrhea, abdominal pain, rash
- **Tapeworms** (Taenia, Diphyllobothrium)
  Obtained Through: undercooked beef, pork, or fish
  Common Symptoms: weight loss, hunger, vitamin deficiencies
- **Giardia**
  Obtained Through: contaminated water
  Common Symptoms: greasy stools, bloating, cramps, nausea
- **Entamoeba histolytica**
  Obtained Through: contaminated food or water
  Common Symptoms: bloody diarrhea, cramping, fatigue
- **Pinworms**
  Obtained Through: hand-to-mouth from surfaces
  Common Symptoms: anal itching, restless sleep, irritability

SKIN / SUBCUTANEOUS TISSUE

- **Cutaneous larva migrans**
  Obtained Through: sand/soil contaminated with animal feces
  Common Symptoms: itchy, winding rash, redness
- **Scabies (mites)**
  Obtained Through: skin-to-skin contact
  Common Symptoms: intense itching, rash, burrows
- **Filarial worms**
  Obtained Through: mosquito or fly bites
  Common Symptoms: swelling, nodules, itching

LUNGS

- **Lung flukes (Paragonimus)** – more common in Asia
  Obtained Through: raw/undercooked crab or crayfish
  Common Symptoms: chronic cough, chest pain, blood-tinged sputum, shortness of breath
- **Ascaris (larval lung migration)**
  Obtained Through: contaminated food or soil
  Common Symptoms: dry cough, wheezing, fever
- **Strongyloides (lung phase)**
  Obtained Through: skin contact with contaminated soil
  Common Symptoms: cough, chest tightness, rash, abdominal pain

BLOOD

- **Malaria (Plasmodium)** – uncommon unless travel-related
  Obtained Through: mosquito bites
  Common Symptoms: fever, chills, sweats, headache, anemia
- **Babesia**
  Obtained Through: tick bites
  Common Symptoms: fatigue, fever, night sweats, joint pain

LIVER

- **Liver flukes (Fasciola, Clonorchis)** – more common in Asia
  Obtained Through: raw aquatic plants or fish
  Common Symptoms: right-side abdominal pain, nausea, jaundice, fatigue

BRAIN / CENTRAL NERVOUS SYSTEM

- **Toxoplasma gondii**
  Obtained Through: undercooked meat, cat feces, contaminated soil
  Common Symptoms: headache, brain fog, fatigue, mood, seizures
- **Neurocysticercosis (tapeworm larvae)**
  Obtained Through: contaminated food or water
  Common Symptoms: seizures, headaches, confusion, nausea

EYES

- **Toxocara (ocular larva migrans)**
  Obtained Through: dog/cat feces in soil
  Common Symptoms: blurred vision, eye pain, light sensitivity

HEART / BLOOD VESSELS

- **Schistosoma (blood flukes)** – more common in Africa
  Obtained Through: contaminated freshwater exposure
  Common Symptoms: fever, fatigue, inflammation of organs

MUSCLES

- **Trichinella spiralis**
  Obtained Through: undercooked pork or wild game
  Common Symptoms: muscle pain, swelling, fever, weakness

REPRODUCTIVE ORGANS

- **Trichomonas vaginalis**
  Obtained Through: sexual contact
  Common Symptoms: discharge, itching, burning, pelvic pain

BONES

- **Hydatid cysts** – more common in Asia and Middle East
  Obtained Through: dog feces exposure
  Common Symptoms: bone pain, fractures, cyst growth

This list is not exhaustive. Many additional organisms exist, particularly in specific regions of the world, rural environments, or areas with limited sanitation and clean water access. The organisms included here represent some of the more frequently discussed and clinically relevant examples, yet they do not encompass every possible parasitic infection.

Symptoms can offer diagnostic clues. However, many parasite-related symptoms overlap with those of other conditions, meaning the presence of a particular symptom does not automatically indicate a parasitic infection. For this reason, proper medical evaluation and appropriate laboratory testing through a qualified healthcare provider are recommended to confirm or rule out a parasitic cause before assuming a diagnosis or beginning treatment.

It is also important to understand that no diagnostic method is perfect. Certain parasites may be difficult to detect depending on life cycle stage, tissue location, or sampling limitations. A single negative test does not always provide a complete picture, which is why clinical judgment, symptom patterns, and professional guidance remain essential.

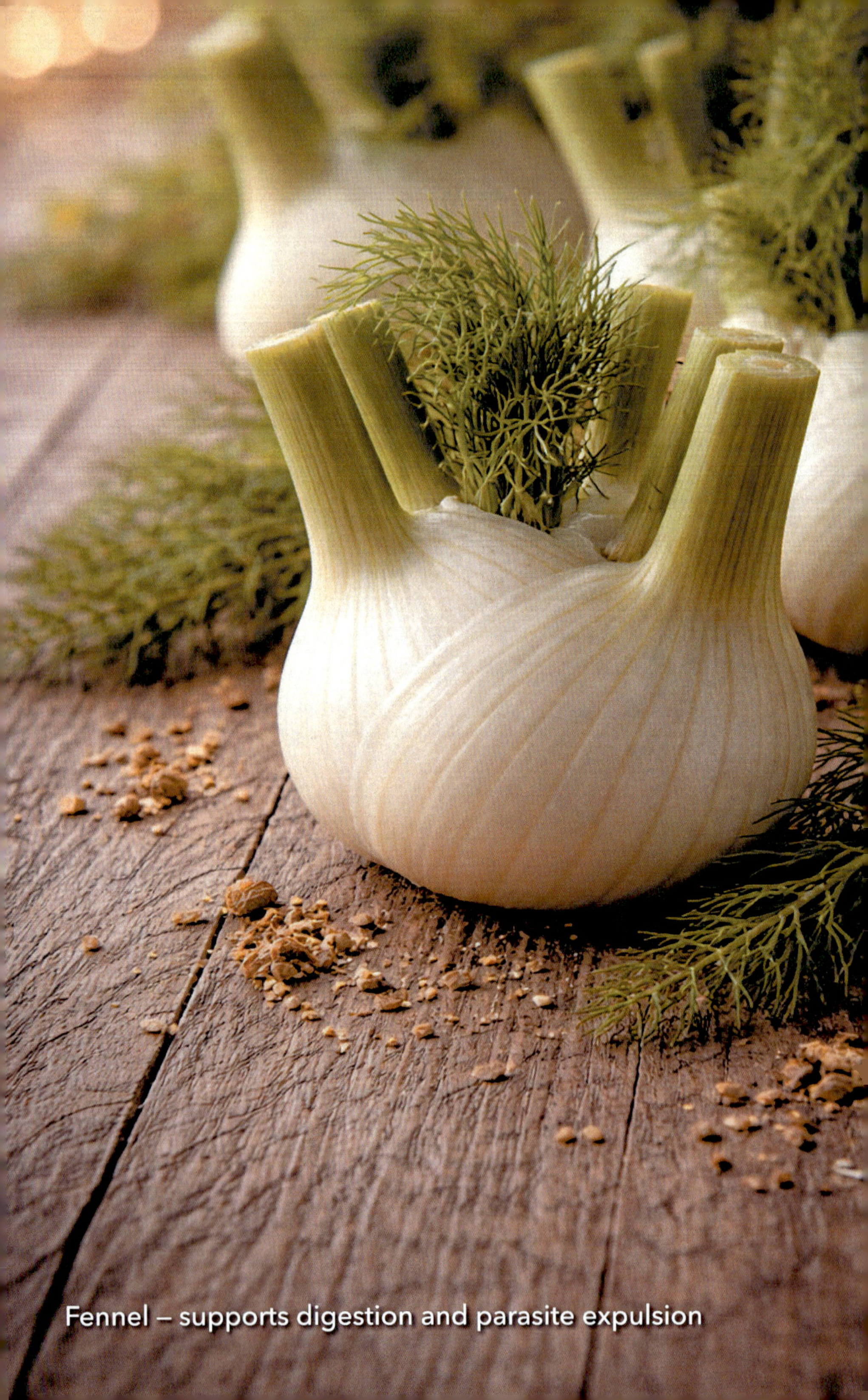

Fennel – supports digestion and parasite expulsion

CHAPTER 2

HOW PARASITES ENTER THE BODY

Unfortunately, parasites do not announce their arrival. They slip in quietly, hitchhiking on everyday habits and ordinary environments. Most people imagine parasites as something you contract only in far-off countries or from extreme, unsanitary conditions. In reality, exposure can happen in modern kitchens, suburban backyards, and even carefully cleaned homes. Understanding how parasites enter the body removes fear and replaces it with awareness and wisdom.

Parasites reach humans through several main pathways: what we eat, what we drink, what we touch, where we travel, and who or what we live with. These routes overlap, meaning exposure is rarely dramatic. It is usually slow, subtle, and cumulative.

FOOD: THE MOST COMMON GATEWAY

Food is one of the most frequent entry points for parasites. Undercooked or raw meat, especially pork, beef, and fish, can harbor microscopic larvae. When meat is not cooked thoroughly, these organisms remain alive and can establish themselves in the digestive tract.

Fresh produce can also be a source. Fruits and vegetables grown in contaminated soil or irrigated with unsafe water may carry parasite eggs. Even organic produce is not immune, because organic farming does not eliminate exposure to wildlife, insects, or contaminated soil. Washing helps, but it does not guarantee complete removal, especially when parasites exist in microscopic forms that cling tightly to surfaces.

Prepared foods can also be contaminated through handling. If someone preparing food carries parasites and does not practice strict hygiene, transmission can occur easily through shared surfaces, utensils, or hands.

WATER: A HIDDEN RISK

Water is another major pathway. Parasites can survive in untreated or poorly treated water supplies, including wells, streams, and even municipal systems when filtration fails. Drinking contaminated water is not the only concern. Parasites can enter through brushing teeth, washing produce, or swallowing water while swimming.

Recreational water sources such as lakes, rivers, and pools may also carry parasites if sanitation is inadequate. Because some parasites are microscopic, water can appear clear and clean while still harboring organisms capable of infecting the body.

PETS AND ANIMALS: CLOSE COMPANIONS, SHARED MICROBES

Domestic pets are loving companions, but they are also common carriers of parasites. Dogs and cats can pick up parasites from soil, other animals, or fleas and bring them directly into the home. Litter boxes, pet bedding, and even fur can transfer parasite eggs to human hands and surfaces.

Children are especially vulnerable because they often play on the floor, touch animals frequently, and put their hands in their mouths. However, adults are not immune. Gardening after pets have used the yard, cleaning litter boxes, or allowing pets to lick faces can all increase exposure.

Wildlife also contributes. Birds, rodents, and insects can introduce parasites into outdoor spaces, which then enter homes through shoes, clothing, or open windows.

TRAVEL: EXPANDING THE EXPOSURE ZONE

Travel increases parasite risk simply by introducing the body to unfamiliar food, water, and environments. Different regions carry different parasite species. Eating local foods, drinking untreated water, or walking barefoot on soil in tropical or rural areas can expose travelers to organisms they have never encountered before.

Even short trips can pose a risk. Hotels, public restrooms, cruise ships, and airplanes involve shared surfaces and close contact with many people. Travel weakens the body's usual defenses by disrupting sleep, digestion, and immune balance, making it easier for parasites to take hold.

SOIL AND THE ENVIRONMENT

Soil is a natural reservoir for parasites. Gardens, sandboxes, and parks can contain parasite eggs deposited by animals or carried by water runoff. Walking barefoot, gardening without gloves, or letting children play in dirt can create direct contact between skin and parasites.

Household dust can also contain parasite eggs tracked in from outdoors. Floors, carpets, and pet areas can become quiet collection points. Regular cleaning reduces risk, but does not eliminate it entirely, especially in homes with pets or frequent outdoor exposure.

PERSON-TO-PERSON TRANSMISSION

Some parasites can easily pass directly from one person to another. This often happens through poor hand hygiene, shared bathrooms, shared bedding, or close physical contact. Daycares, schools, nursing homes, and households are common transmission zones. One infected person can unknowingly spread parasites to others through shared surfaces or food preparation. Because many parasites cause mild or vague symptoms at first, people may carry and spread them without realizing it.

WHY EVEN "CLEAN" PEOPLE CAN BE AFFECTED

A common myth is that parasites only affect people who live in dirty conditions. Clean homes, filtered water, and good hygiene reduce risk, but they do not eliminate exposure. Parasites are part of the natural world. They exist in soil, animals, water, and food systems, even in developed countries.

Being "clean" does not mean being isolated from nature. People who eat fresh produce, garden, travel, own pets, or spend time outdoors are constantly interacting with environments where parasites live. Modern life also introduces new risks through mass food distribution, global travel, and densely populated living spaces.

Another factor is immune stress. Poor sleep, chronic stress, nutritional deficiencies, and toxin exposure can weaken the body's natural defenses. A parasite that might normally be eliminated can instead survive and multiply when the internal terrain is compromised.

AWARENESS AS THE FIRST LINE OF DEFENSE

Knowing how parasites enter the body changes how we view prevention. It shifts the focus from fear to stewardship of health. Washing produce thoroughly, cooking meat properly, supporting digestive and immune function, and practicing good hygiene are not acts of paranoia. They are acts of wisdom.

Parasites do not discriminate. They exploit opportunity. The goal is not to live in fear of exposure, but to understand that exposure is possible for everyone. This understanding lays the foundation for why periodic cleansing, vigilance, and strengthening the body's internal environment become important topics in the chapters ahead.

In the next chapter, we will explore the most common parasites that affect humans, how they behave inside the body, and why their symptoms are often mistaken for other conditions.

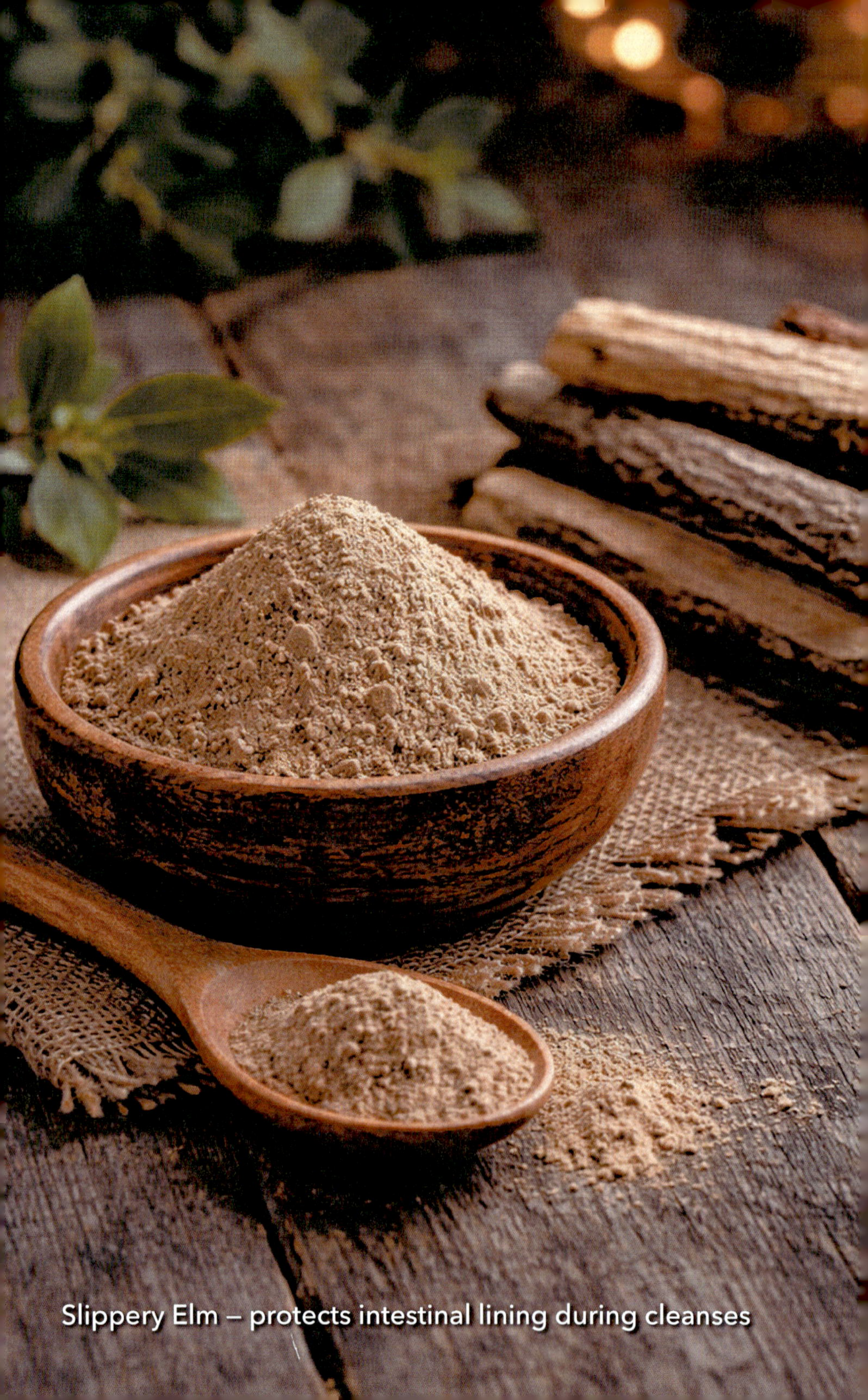

Slippery Elm – protects intestinal lining during cleanses

CHAPTER 3
SIGNS & SYMPTOMS

SIGNS AND SYMPTOMS OF PARASITIC BURDEN

Parasites are masters of disguise. They rarely announce themselves plainly, and they almost never come with a neat label saying, "I'm the problem." Instead, they show up as scattered, stubborn symptoms that don't quite fit into a clean diagnosis. Many people live for years with unresolved health issues, treating surface symptoms while the deeper cause goes unnoticed.

A parasitic burden does not mean someone is dirty, careless, or unhealthy by nature. Exposure can happen through food, water, pets, soil, travel, and even routine daily life. Both exposure and your terrain (the condition of your body) are important factors that determine whether parasites take hold. When digestion is weak, detox pathways are sluggish, or immune function is compromised, parasites can find opportunity. Understanding the symptoms and patterns is one of the most important steps in identifying whether parasites may be contributing to chronic or mysterious health struggles.

DIGESTIVE SYMPTOMS

The digestive system is the most common place for parasites to settle, so gut symptoms are often the first and loudest signals. Common digestive complaints linked to parasitic burden include bloating that does not respond to dietary changes, gas that seems excessive or foul-smelling, alternating diarrhea and constipation, and persistent abdominal discomfort. Some people experience nausea or a sensation of movement or fluttering in the gut, especially at night when the body is still.

Another common sign is sudden or unexplained food sensitivities. Foods that were once tolerated may begin to cause discomfort, inflammation, or digestive upset. Cravings can also become intense, particularly for sugar and refined carbohydrates. Parasites thrive on glucose, and their presence can influence appetite and blood sugar patterns.

Weight changes may occur in either direction. Some individuals struggle to gain weight despite eating regularly, while others experience stubborn weight gain that does not respond to diet or exercise. Malabsorption can develop when parasites interfere with nutrient uptake, leading to deficiencies even when food intake seems adequate.

SKIN, SLEEP, AND NEUROLOGICAL SYMPTOMS

The skin often reflects what is happening internally. Rashes, itching, eczema-like patches, unexplained hives, and chronic acne can all be linked to toxic burden in the body. Nighttime itching, especially around the nose or rectal area, has long been associated with parasitic activity, particularly in children, but also in adults.

Sleep disturbances are another frequent clue. Many people with parasitic burden report difficulty falling asleep, waking between 1:00 and 3:00 a.m., or experiencing vivid or disturbing dreams. This timing is not random. It often overlaps with liver detoxification cycles, when both toxins and organisms may become more active.

Neurological symptoms can be subtle or severe. These may include brain fog, difficulty concentrating, irritability, anxiety, restlessness, or unexplained mood swings. Some individuals report tingling sensations, muscle twitching, or headaches with no clear cause. Because parasites release metabolic waste products, their presence can increase the body's toxic load, affecting nervous system signaling and clarity of thought.

IMMUNE AND INFLAMMATORY EFFECTS

Parasites place constant demand on immune function. Over time, this sustained activation can promote chronic inflammatory signaling or gradual immune exhaustion. Regulatory pathways that normally maintain balance may become strained, altering how the body responds to both internal and external stressors. Instead of responding with precision, the immune system may shift toward patterns of overactivation or diminished responsiveness.

Frequent infections, lingering colds, or slow recovery from illness can reflect immune strain. Allergies and sensitivities may intensify as inflammatory mediators remain elevated and vigilance stays high. Joint discomfort, muscle aches, skin flares, and generalized inflammatory symptoms may surface without a clear mechanical cause, reflecting systemic immune burden rather than localized injury.

Autoimmune-like patterns sometimes emerge, where the body appears to be reacting against its own tissues. In some cases, this represents disrupted immune regulation rather than classical autoimmune disease. Chronic antigen exposure, endotoxin circulation, and persistent organism presence can distort signaling pathways that govern tolerance and defense. The immune system continually works to distinguish between self and invader, and parasitic burden complicates that discernment, increasing the risk of misdirected or prolonged inflammatory responses.

WHEN SYMPTOMS MIMIC OTHER CONDITIONS

One of the greatest challenges with parasitic burden is that the symptoms often look like something else. Digestive issues may be labeled as irritable bowel syndrome. Fatigue may be called adrenal burnout. Brain fog may be attributed to stress or aging. Skin eruptions may be treated as purely dermatological.

The symptom pattern can feel scattered and unrelated because parasites affect multiple systems at once. A person may be treated by different specialists for different complaints without ever addressing the root cause.

This is why parasitic burden is frequently overlooked. Modern medicine tends to separate the body into compartments, while parasites operate system-wide. When symptoms do not respond to standard treatments, it may be time to look deeper rather than to simply try a new medication or protocol.

WHY STANDARD TESTING OFTEN MISSES THEM

Conventional stool testing is designed to detect specific organisms, usually in advanced or acute infections. Many parasites do not shed eggs or detectable markers consistently. Some hide in tissues rather than remaining in the intestinal tract. Others exist in life stages that evade routine testing methods.

False negatives are common. A single negative test does not necessarily rule out parasitic involvement, especially when symptom patterns strongly suggest it. Testing also depends heavily on timing, sample handling, and laboratory techniques.

Additionally, many people carry low-grade parasitic loads rather than overt infestations. These burdens may not show up clearly on lab work but can still produce chronic symptoms over time.

For this reason, symptom assessment, exposure history, and clinical patterns become just as important as laboratory data. The body often tells the story before the test ever does.

Parasites do not always create dramatic illness overnight. More often, they quietly drain vitality, disrupt digestion, confuse immune responses, and cloud mental clarity. Recognizing the signs is more about awareness than fear. When patterns are understood, action can be taken thoughtfully and responsibly.

In the next chapter, we will explore the body's detoxification system and how parasites can interfere with detox pathways.

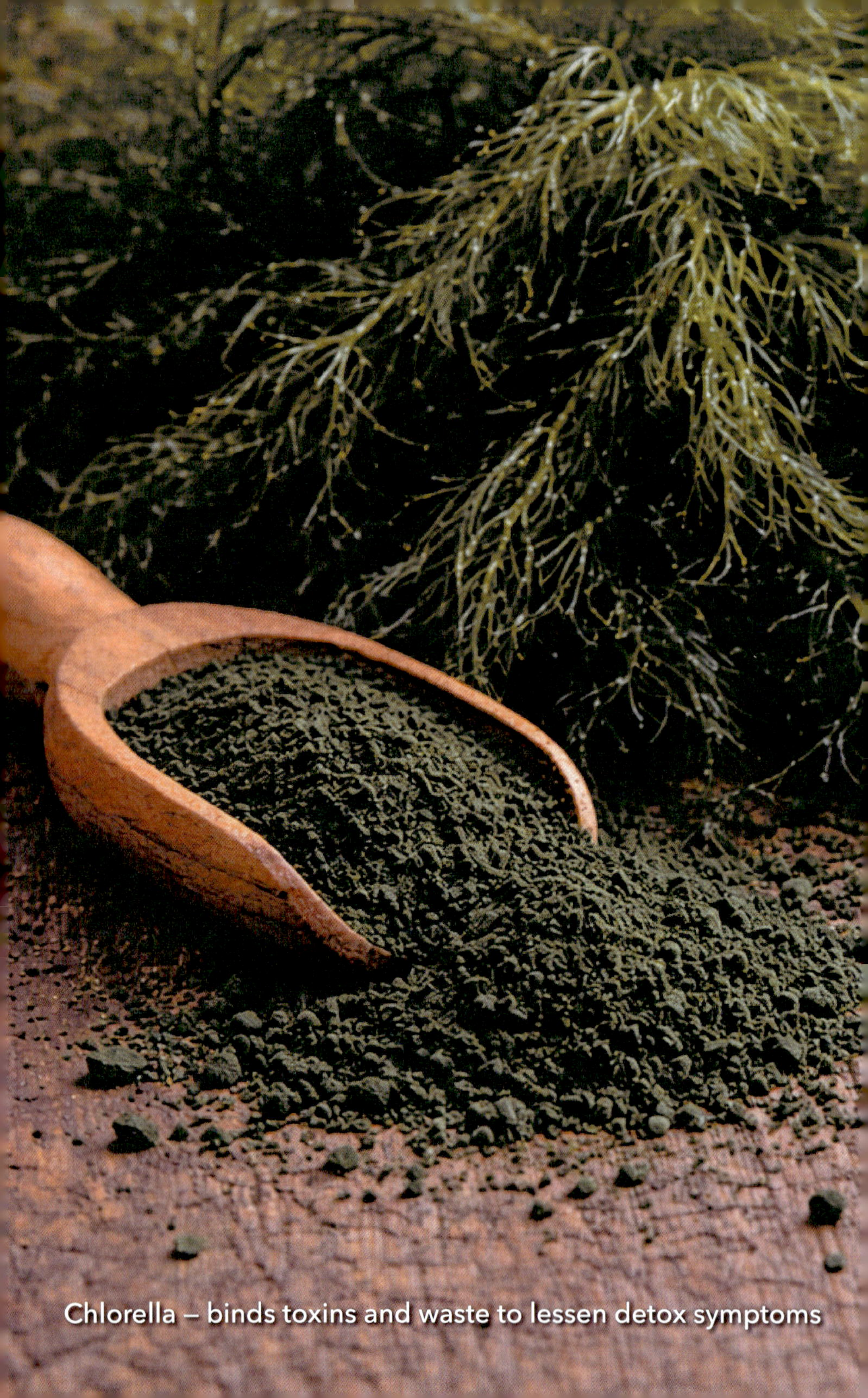

Chlorella – binds toxins and waste to lessen detox symptoms

CHAPTER 4
DETOX PATHWAYS

THE BODY'S DETOXIFICATION SYSTEMS

Your body was designed by God with built-in systems of cleansing and renewal. Every day, without you consciously directing it, your body filters blood, neutralizes toxins, moves waste, and eliminates what does not belong. Detoxification is a God-given process woven into human physiology. When these systems are supported, the body can handle a surprising toxic load. When they are overwhelmed or obstructed, toxins accumulate, inflammation rises, and symptoms appear. Parasites thrive in exactly these conditions.

The goal of a parasite cleanse is not simply to kill parasites. The goal is to restore proper flow through the body's elimination channels so waste can leave efficiently and safely. Detoxification depends on five primary pathways working together: the liver, gallbladder, kidneys, lymphatic system, and gastrointestinal tract.

THE LIVER: THE MASTER DETOXIFIER

The liver is the body's primary filtration organ. Every drop of blood from the digestive tract passes through it before entering general circulation. Its role is to neutralize toxins, break down chemicals, metabolize hormones, and prepare waste for removal.

When parasites are present, the liver becomes burdened in several ways. Parasites release metabolic waste, ammonia, and neurotoxins as part of their life cycle. Many also produce substances that suppress immune detection, further stressing liver function. Over time, this toxic load slows the liver's detox pathways, making it harder to process both internal waste and external toxins from food, air, and medications.

A sluggish liver affects digestion, impacts energy levels, hormone balance, blood sugar regulation, and mental clarity. Supporting liver detoxification is foundational before aggressive parasite killing begins.

THE GALLBLADDER: THE FAT AND WASTE TRANSPORTER

The gallbladder stores and releases bile, a substance produced by the liver. Bile plays a critical role in digesting fats and carrying fat-soluble toxins out of the body through the intestines.

Parasites commonly interfere with bile flow. Some organisms physically inhabit bile ducts, while others thicken bile through inflammation and toxic byproducts. When bile becomes sluggish, toxins continue to be recirculated in the body instead of being eliminated.

Poor bile flow often presents as bloating, constipation, pale stools, nausea after fatty meals, or right-sided abdominal discomfort. Without adequate bile movement, detoxification slows and parasite waste accumulates.

THE KIDNEYS: THE BLOOD FILTERS

The kidneys filter blood continuously, removing water-soluble toxins and maintaining proper electrolyte balance. They rely on hydration and mineral balance to perform this task effectively.

During a parasite cleanse, kidney burden increases because more toxins are being mobilized for elimination. If kidney filtration is compromised or hydration is inadequate, toxins remain circulating in the bloodstream. This can lead to headaches, fatigue, muscle aches, and dizziness. Supporting kidney function through hydration and gentle detox support allows the body to remove waste without overwhelming the system.

THE LYMPHATIC SYSTEM: THE WASTE TRANSPORT NETWORK

The lymphatic system functions as the body's drainage network. It collects cellular waste, immune debris, and toxins from tissues and transports them toward elimination. Unlike the heart-driven circulatory system, lymph relies on movement, breathing, and muscle contraction to flow.

Parasites contribute to lymph stagnation by triggering chronic immune activation and inflammation. Thickened lymph slows detoxification and allows toxins to remain stored in tissues. This can manifest as swollen glands, chronic congestion, body aches, and persistent fatigue. Without proper lymph movement, detoxification becomes incomplete even if the liver and kidneys are functioning well.

THE GUT: THE FINAL EXIT PATHWAY

The digestive tract is the final elimination route for much of the body's toxic waste. Bile carries toxins into the intestines, and healthy bowel movements ensure they leave the body rather than being reabsorbed.

Parasites disrupt gut integrity by damaging the intestinal lining, altering microbiome balance, and producing substances that increase permeability. This allows toxins to leak back into circulation instead of exiting through stool.

Constipation during a parasite cleanse is uncomfortable and dangerous. When waste does not leave the body, detoxification reverses direction and becomes re-toxification.

HOW PARASITES INTERFERE WITH DETOX PATHWAYS

Parasites survive by manipulating their environment. They block bile flow, inflame tissues, suppress immune responses, and produce toxic waste that weakens detox organs. Their presence creates congestion within the very systems meant to remove them.

As parasites die, they release stored toxins, heavy metals, and metabolic debris. If detox pathways are not open and functioning, these toxins accumulate in circulation. This is what creates severe cleansing reactions rather than healing responses. Parasite cleansing without drainage is like demolishing a building without hauling away the rubble.

WHY ELIMINATION IS JUST AS IMPORTANT AS KILLING

Many protocols focus on attacking parasites but neglect elimination. Killing without clearing creates a toxic traffic jam inside the body. The result is overload rather than restoration. True cleansing occurs when the body can process and remove waste efficiently. This means bowel regularity, bile flow, hydration, lymph movement, and liver support must be addressed alongside antiparasitic strategies. Elimination is equal in importance to eradication. Without it, even effective parasite-killing herbs or compounds can make symptoms worse instead of better.

THE DANGER OF "DIE-OFF" WITHOUT DRAINAGE

Die-off reactions occur when large numbers of organisms are killed rapidly and release toxins faster than the body can eliminate them. Symptoms may include headaches, nausea, skin eruptions, fatigue, brain fog, anxiety, joint pain, and flu-like sensations.

While some mild discomfort may occur during cleansing, intense reactions are not a sign of success. They are a sign of congestion. The body is overwhelmed by waste that cannot exit. Proper drainage reduces these reactions and protects vital organs from toxin overload. This is why a parasite cleanse must always support the detoxification systems first and throughout the process.

God designed the body to cleanse itself. Our role is not to force detoxification, but to restore flow. When elimination pathways are open, the body can do what it was created to do: remove what does not belong and restore what was compromised.

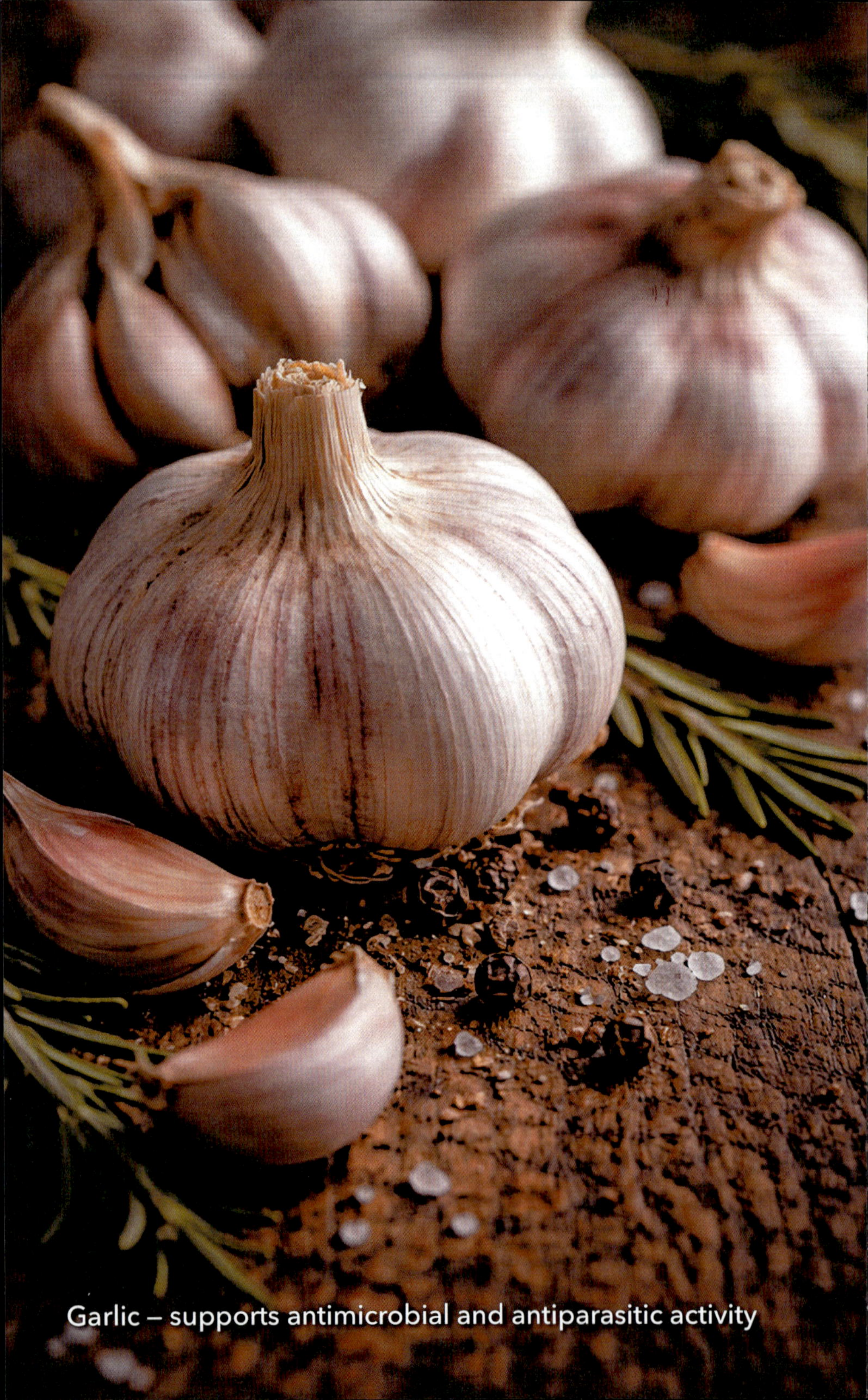

Garlic – supports antimicrobial and antiparasitic activity

CHAPTER 5
THE MICROBIOME

THE MICROBIOME AND PARASITES

Inside the human digestive tract lives a complex ecosystem made up of trillions of microorganisms. This community, known as the microbiome, plays a central role in digestion, immune signaling, nutrient absorption, and protection against unwanted invaders. When this ecosystem is balanced, it behaves like a well-organized city with clear boundaries and strong defenses. When it becomes disrupted, space opens up for organisms that do not belong there.

Parasites do not arrive in an empty environment. They enter a living system already populated by bacteria, yeasts, and immune cells. The condition of that system largely determines whether they pass through or take hold.

RELATIONSHIP BETWEEN PARASITES AND GUT FLORA

Parasites and gut flora exist in constant interaction. Some parasites compete directly with beneficial bacteria for nutrients. Others alter the environment of the gut by producing metabolic waste that changes pH and weakens protective barriers. Over time, this shifts the internal terrain in their favor.

Instead of being quickly removed, parasites find conditions that allow them to persist. They may interfere with bile flow or digestive enzymes, reducing the body's ability to fully break down food. Undigested material then feeds imbalanced microbes, further altering the microbiome. This creates a biological setting that supports survival rather than elimination of the unwanted parasites.

HOW DYSBIOSIS ALLOWS OVERGROWTH

A healthy microbiome functions as a line of resistance. Beneficial bacteria occupy attachment sites along the intestinal lining and help prevent harmful organisms from gaining a foothold. They also produce compounds that discourage the growth of unwanted microbes and support the production of protective mucus.

When dysbiosis develops, resistance weakens. Dysbiosis refers to an imbalance in the microbial community, often marked by reduced diversity and overgrowth of opportunistic organisms. Antibiotic use, chronic stress, poor diet, environmental toxins, and repeated infections can all contribute to this shift.

With fewer good bacteria present, parasites encounter less competition and more available resources. The gut becomes more permeable, inflammation increases, and immune signaling becomes less precise. Instead of responding efficiently, the system grows confused and reactive. This allows organisms that would normally be kept in check to multiply.

Once established, parasites can drive dysbiosis even further. Their waste products irritate tissue and alter the chemical environment of the gut. This creates a reinforcing cycle in which dysbiosis supports parasites and parasites deepen dysbiosis.

THE ROLE OF BENEFICIAL BACTERIA IN RESISTANCE

Beneficial bacteria help regulate inflammation and support the integrity of the intestinal lining. They strengthen tight junctions, assist immune cells in recognizing threats, and influence how antigens (foreign threats) are presented to the immune system. In this way, they shape both physical and immune defenses.

A well-supported microbiome does not eliminate parasites on its own, but it improves the body's ability to resist colonization and recover faster after exposure. It creates an environment that is less favorable for invaders and more supportive of balanced immune response.

Beneficial bacteria function as part of a coordinated system that reinforces the gut barrier and reduces opportunities for overgrowth.

WHY REBUILDING THE GUT IS ESSENTIAL AFTER DETOX

Removing parasites without restoring the terrain leaves the system vulnerable to reinfection and imbalance. The environment that allowed overgrowth in the first place must be changed.

Post-detox gut rebuilding is a phase of stabilization. It allows the body to reclaim space that may have been occupied by parasites or opportunistic organisms. It also helps normalize immune communication so the system does not remain locked in irritation or hypervigilance.

Rebuilding involves nourishing beneficial bacteria, repairing the intestinal lining, and supporting digestive secretions so food is fully broken down rather than becoming fuel for unwanted microbes. This shift reduces the likelihood that future exposures will take hold.

The microbiome is influenced by sleep, hydration, stress hormones, and food choices. A detox protocol may reduce a burden, but long-term resilience depends on what is built afterward. The goal is balance.

Parasites thrive in disrupted ecosystems. A healthy microbiome makes their survival more difficult. By restoring bacterial diversity and strengthening gut integrity after detoxification, the body moves from vulnerability toward resistance. This is not merely cleanup after a protocol. It is the foundation that determines whether progress is temporary or lasting.

In the larger picture, parasite cleansing and microbiome restoration function as two parts of the same strategy. One reduces the burden. The other rebuilds the defense. Without both, the system remains incomplete.

Rebuilding the microbiome is not only about what is removed, but also about what is reintroduced. Daily contact with the natural world helps restore microbial diversity that modern life has reduced.

SIMPLE WAYS TO SUPPORT BENEFICIAL GUT BACTERIA

- Eat a wide variety of whole foods, herbs, and natural fibers
- Rotate foods instead of eating the same meals every day
- Spend time outdoors in natural environments
- Garden or handle soil occasionally without gloves
- Walk barefoot on grass, sand, or natural ground when safe
- Interact with pets and animals (petting, normal affection)
- Avoid unnecessary overuse of antibacterial soaps and sanitizers
- Reduce highly processed and ultra-refined foods
- Support regular digestion and elimination
- Prioritize sleep and stress regulation
- For infants, vaginal birth and breastfeeding help establish a healthy foundational microbiome
- Use rotating probiotic blends rather than relying on a single product
- Consume fermented foods when tolerated (such as sauerkraut, kefir, yogurt, kimchi, or pickled vegetables)
- Eat prebiotic foods (non-digestible fibers that feed good bacteria): include onions, garlic, leeks, asparagus, and Jerusalem artichokes
- Eat resistant starches such as cooled potatoes or green bananas
- Chew food thoroughly to support microbial breakdown
- Maintain regular bowel elimination so waste does not stagnate

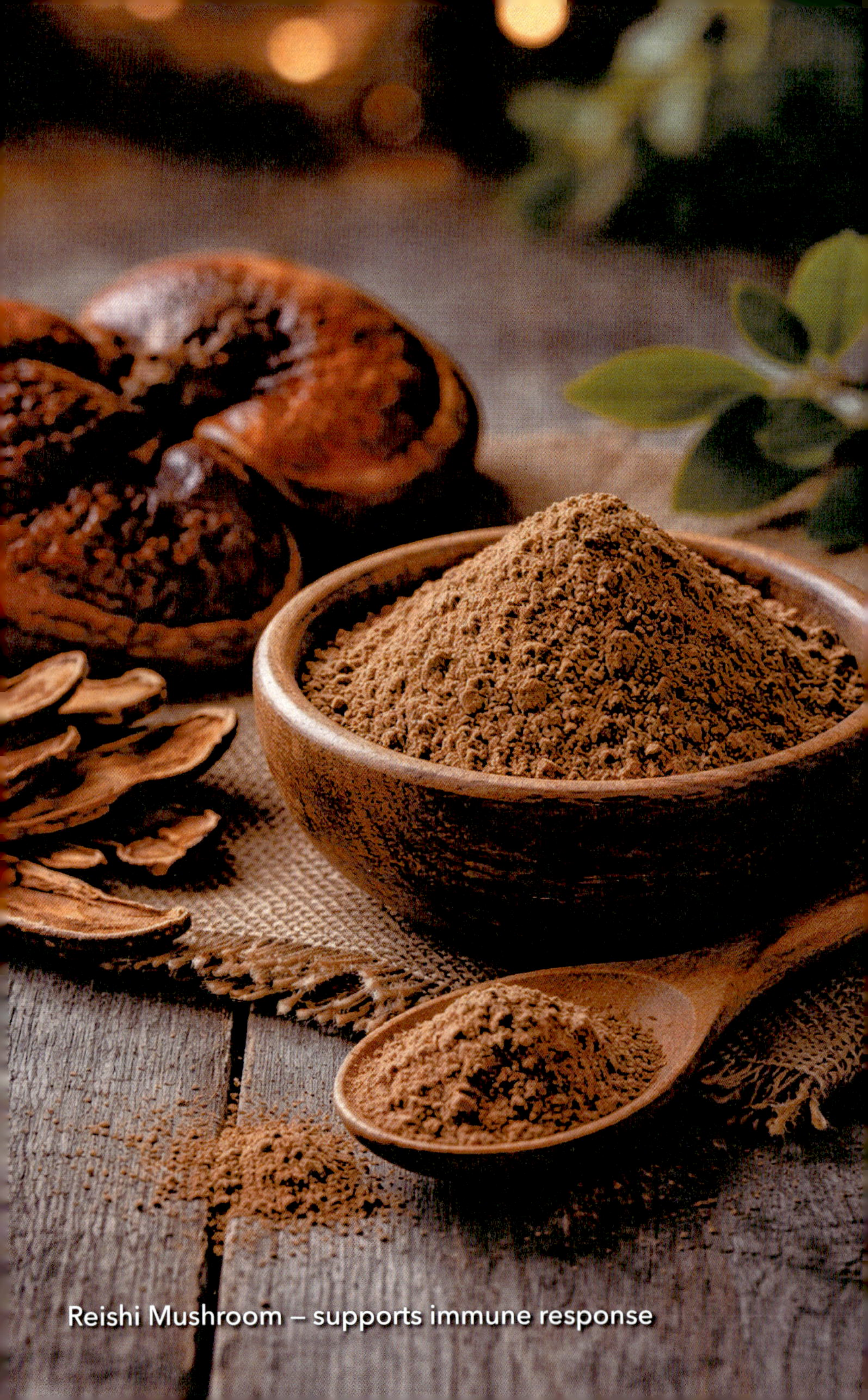

Reishi Mushroom – supports immune response

CHAPTER 6
NUTRITION

NUTRITION FOR PARASITE DETOXIFICATION

Every meal either strengthens the body's terrain or feeds the problem it is trying to resolve. During parasite detoxification, nutrition becomes a form of strategy. Certain foods support the liver, gut, and immune system so the body can remove waste efficiently. Other foods create an internal environment that parasites prefer.

FOODS THAT SUPPORT DETOXIFICATION PATHWAYS

The liver, gallbladder, kidneys, lymphatic system, and gut rely on specific nutrients to do their work. Whole, unprocessed foods supply those nutrients in a form the body recognizes.

Detoxification foods include:

- Cruciferous vegetables such as broccoli, cauliflower, cabbage, and Brussels sprouts, which support liver enzyme activity
- Leafy greens such as spinach, arugula, and parsley, which support bile flow and mineral balance
- Sulfur-rich foods such as garlic, onions, and leeks, which assist Phase II liver detoxification
- Bitter foods such as dandelion greens and radicchio, which stimulate digestive secretions
- Fermented foods such as sauerkraut and kimchi, which help rebuild beneficial gut bacteria
- Herbs and spices such as turmeric, ginger, and oregano, which support inflammation control and microbial balance

These foods do not "kill" parasites on their own. They strengthen the systems responsible for elimination so the body can handle what is released during cleansing.

FOODS PARASITES THRIVE ON

Parasites favor environments that are rich in quick energy and low in immune resistance. Diets built around refined carbohydrates and highly processed foods create ideal conditions for overgrowth.

Foods that commonly support parasite survival include:

- Sugars and syrups
- Refined flours and baked goods
- Sweetened beverages and fruit juices

- Ultra-processed snacks
- Alcohol
- Excessive starches without fiber

These foods spike blood sugar, disrupt gut flora, and weaken immune signaling. Over time, they shift the terrain toward imbalance. Removing them does not starve parasites instantly, but it reduces their advantage while supporting the body's defenses.

PROTEIN, FATS, AND FIBER BALANCE

Macronutrients each play a specific role in detoxification and recovery.

Protein

Protein supplies amino acids needed for liver enzymes, immune cells, and tissue repair. Without enough protein, detoxification can stall because the body lacks the building blocks required for processing waste.

Good sources of protein include:

- Eggs
- Poultry
- Beef or lamb
- Fish
- Bone broth

Fats

Healthy fats support bile production and hormone signaling. They also provide steady energy so blood sugar remains stable during cleansing.

Helpful fats include:

- Olive oil
- Avocado
- Coconut oil
- Butter or ghee
- Fatty fish

Fiber

Fiber binds waste in the intestines and supports regular elimination. It also feeds beneficial bacteria that compete with harmful organisms.

Fiber sources include:

- Vegetables
- Seeds
- Berries
- Ground flax or chia

A balanced intake of protein, fats, and fiber prevents detox symptoms from escalating due to weakness, blood sugar swings, or constipation.

HYDRATION AND MINERAL SUPPORT

Detoxification increases the body's demand for fluids. Water is the transport system for waste removal through the kidneys, lymphatic system, and bowels. Hydration should be consistent throughout the day rather than consumed in large amounts at once.

In addition to water, minerals are essential. Sodium, potassium, magnesium, and trace minerals support nerve signaling, muscle function, and cellular transport. Without them, fatigue, dizziness, and headaches are more likely.

Helpful hydration options include:

- Mineral-rich water
- Homemade broths
- Electrolyte blends without added sugar
- Herbal teas

FASTING AND TIMING CONSIDERATIONS (Optional)

Some people choose to use fasting or meal timing as part of parasite detoxification. Fasting is not required for a parasite cleanse.

Short fasting windows or extended overnight breaks from eating may:

- Improve insulin sensitivity
- Increase digestive rest
- Encourage cellular cleanup
- Reduce constant glucose supply

However, fasting should never lead to weakness, dizziness, or nutrient depletion. For some individuals, stable meals with adequate protein and minerals are more supportive than food restriction.

PUTTING IT ALL TOGETHER

Nutrition during parasite detoxification supports an internal environment that favors healing rather than survival of unwanted organisms. When food supports detoxification pathways, parasites lose their advantage. The terrain shifts. Elimination becomes more efficient. Symptoms are more manageable. Recovery is more complete.

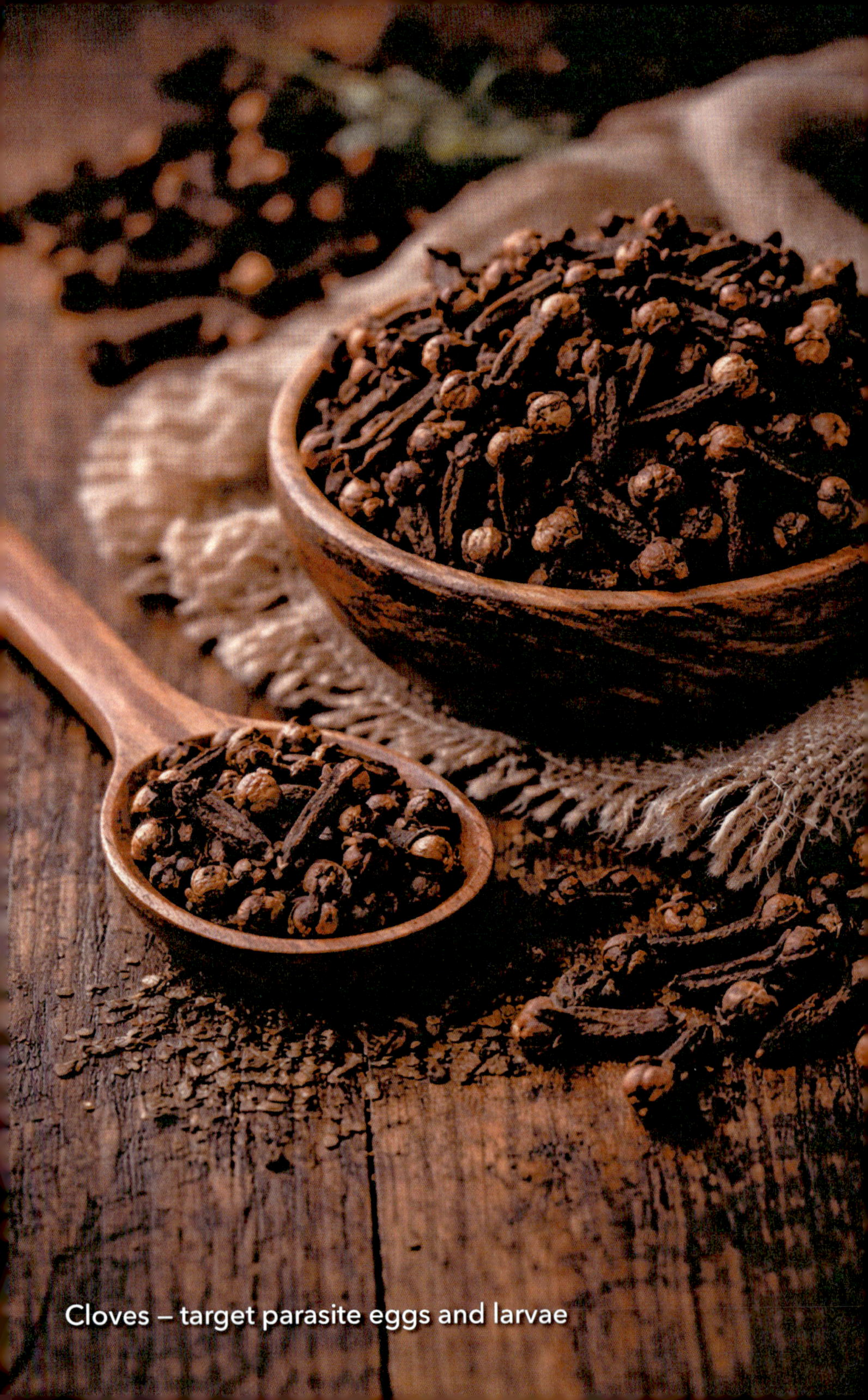

Cloves – target parasite eggs and larvae

CHAPTER 7

NATURAL PARASITE ELIMINATORS

TARGETED TOOLS, WISE USE, STEADY STRATEGY

Natural anti-parasitic agents have been used across cultures for centuries. Traditional herbal systems, modern phytochemistry, and emerging research all point to the same truth: certain plants and compounds can help create an intestinal environment that is hostile to unwanted organisms and supportive of host resilience. Natural agents work best when they are combined wisely, rotated intentionally, and supported by nutrition, elimination, and immune function.

HERBS TRADITIONALLY USED FOR PARASITES

Many anti-parasitic herbs come from traditional systems such as Ayurveda, Traditional Chinese Medicine (TCM), and European Herbalism. Their historical use often aligns with modern findings on antimicrobial, antiparasitic, and digestive-supportive compounds.

Commonly used herbs include:

Clove

- Traditionally used to target parasite eggs and larvae
- Rich in eugenol and other phenolic compounds
- Often paired with other herbs rather than used alone

Wormwood

- Historically used for intestinal worms
- Bitter compounds support digestive secretions
- Often included in classic parasite formulas

Black Walnut Hull

- Traditionally used for intestinal cleansing
- Contains juglone and tannins
- Commonly paired with clove and wormwood in classic triads

Garlic

- Broad spectrum antimicrobial activity
- Supports microbial balance
- Also supports cardiovascular and immune function

Neem
- Widely used in Ayurvedic practice
- Supports antimicrobial and antiparasitic defense
- Often used in rotation due to potency

Thyme and Oregano
- Strong aromatic herbs
- Contain volatile oils with antimicrobial activity
- More often used as extracts or oils than teas

Mugwort
- Traditional digestive and expulsion herb
- Same plant family as wormwood
- Historically used in parasite protocols

Holarrhena
- Used traditionally for intestinal infections and dysentery patterns
- Studied for activity against certain protozoal organisms

BOTANICAL COMPOUNDS AND ESSENTIAL OILS

Plants produce protective chemicals to defend themselves. Many of these compounds show antimicrobial or antiparasitic activity in laboratory and clinical settings.

Phenols and phenolic acids
- Found in clove, oregano, thyme
- Membrane-disruptive to microbes in lab models

Terpenes and terpenoids
- Found in wormwood, neem, many aromatic herbs
- Often bitter and biologically active

Alkaloids
- Present in several traditional antiparasitic plants
- Often potent and dose-sensitive

Essential oils
- Highly concentrated plant extracts
- Examples include oregano oil, thyme oil, clove oil
- Show strong antimicrobial activity in vitro

SUPPORTIVE SUPPLEMENTS

Not all helpful agents directly target parasites. Some strengthen host defenses, digestive function, and elimination pathways. These are force multipliers (increases the effectiveness of the main force).

Berberine-containing plants

- Found in barberry and goldenseal
- Studied for antimicrobial and protozoal effects
- Also supports metabolic and gut barrier function

Caprylic acid

- Fatty acid found in coconut
- Supports microbial balance
- Often used in yeast and dysbiosis protocols

Pumpkin seed

- Traditionally used for intestinal worms
- Compounds may interfere with parasite attachment and motility
- Gentle and food-based

Papaya seed

- Traditional expulsion agent
- Enzyme and alkaloid content
- Often used short term

Digestive enzymes

- Support protein breakdown
- May help disrupt biofilms and protective coatings
- Support overall digestion and nutrient absorption

Probiotics

- Support microbial balance and competitive exclusion
- Help reinforce gut barrier integrity
- Support immune regulation during and after antimicrobial phases

Prebiotics

- Provide fermentable fibers that nourish beneficial bacteria
- Support short-chain fatty acid production
- Help restore microbial diversity after disruption

Minerals and trace elements

- Zinc and selenium support immune function
- Copper supports immune cell development and function
- Magnesium supports elimination
- Electrolytes support hydration and bowel regularity

BINDING AGENTS

Binding agents catch and carry out the trash. When organisms are damaged or killed, they release cellular debris and metabolic byproducts. Binding agents help capture unwanted compounds in the gut so they can be eliminated rather than reabsorbed.

Activated charcoal

- High-surface area absorption
- Binds toxins and microbial byproducts
- Must be spaced away from medications and nutrients

Herb binders

- Chlorella and cilantro
- Chlorella acts as a gentle binder support in the gut
- Cilantro is more of a mobilizer and is best paired with binders
- Bind toxins and microbial byproducts
- Must be spaced away from medications and nutrients

Clay minerals

- Bentonite and other clays
- Absorptive capacity
- Traditionally used for gastrointestinal distress

Fiber blends

- Soluble and insoluble fibers
- Support bowel motility
- Feed beneficial microbes when chosen wisely

Algae-based binders

- Certain algae compounds bind unwanted substances
- Also support elimination

Key principles:

- Use binders away from supplements and medications
- Maintain hydration
- Support daily bowel movements
- Adjust dose to tolerance
- No exit pathway means recirculation – elimination is essential

WHY ROTATION AND COMBINATION MATTER

Different herbs and compounds work through distinct mechanisms of action. Some demonstrate greater activity against egg stages, while others are more effective against active or adult forms. Certain botanicals disrupt cellular membranes, others interfere with metabolic processes, and others alter the terrain of the gut environment. Using a thoughtful combination allows these mechanisms to work synergistically rather than relying on a single biological pathway. Rotation may also help limit biological tolerance that can develop with continuous exposure to one dominant mechanism, while potentially reducing side effects associated with prolonged, uninterrupted dosing.

Another important consideration is the life cycle rhythm of many parasites. Organisms do not remain in a single uniform state. They hatch, mature, migrate, reproduce, encyst, and in some cases enter dormant phases before reactivating. Strategic rotation accounts for these biological shifts rather than assuming a static target. By periodically adjusting pressure and mechanism, the protocol remains responsive rather than predictable, which may improve overall reduction without unnecessarily escalating intensity.

Strategic rotation also creates physiological breathing room. Antimicrobial pressure increases antigen exposure and immune signaling as organisms break down. When pressure is continuous and unrelenting, inflammatory mediators and oxidative demand may accumulate in susceptible individuals. Intentional pauses allow cytokine signaling to settle, oxidative stress to normalize, and elimination pathways to catch up with mobilized debris. More intensity is not always more effective. Intelligent sequencing respects the body's capacity to process what is being mobilized while preserving forward progress.

In practice, combination strategy often means pairing agents that address multiple vulnerabilities simultaneously. This may include supporting the targeting of egg stages alongside active stages, or combining membrane disruptors with metabolic inhibitors. Direct antiparasitic agents are also best paired with binders and elimination support so that debris and metabolic byproducts are efficiently carried out rather than recirculated.

Typical rotation patterns use a combination for two to four weeks, followed by a short break, then a new combination or adjusted ratios before repeating another cycle if needed. The goal of a successful parasite detox is intelligent sequencing.

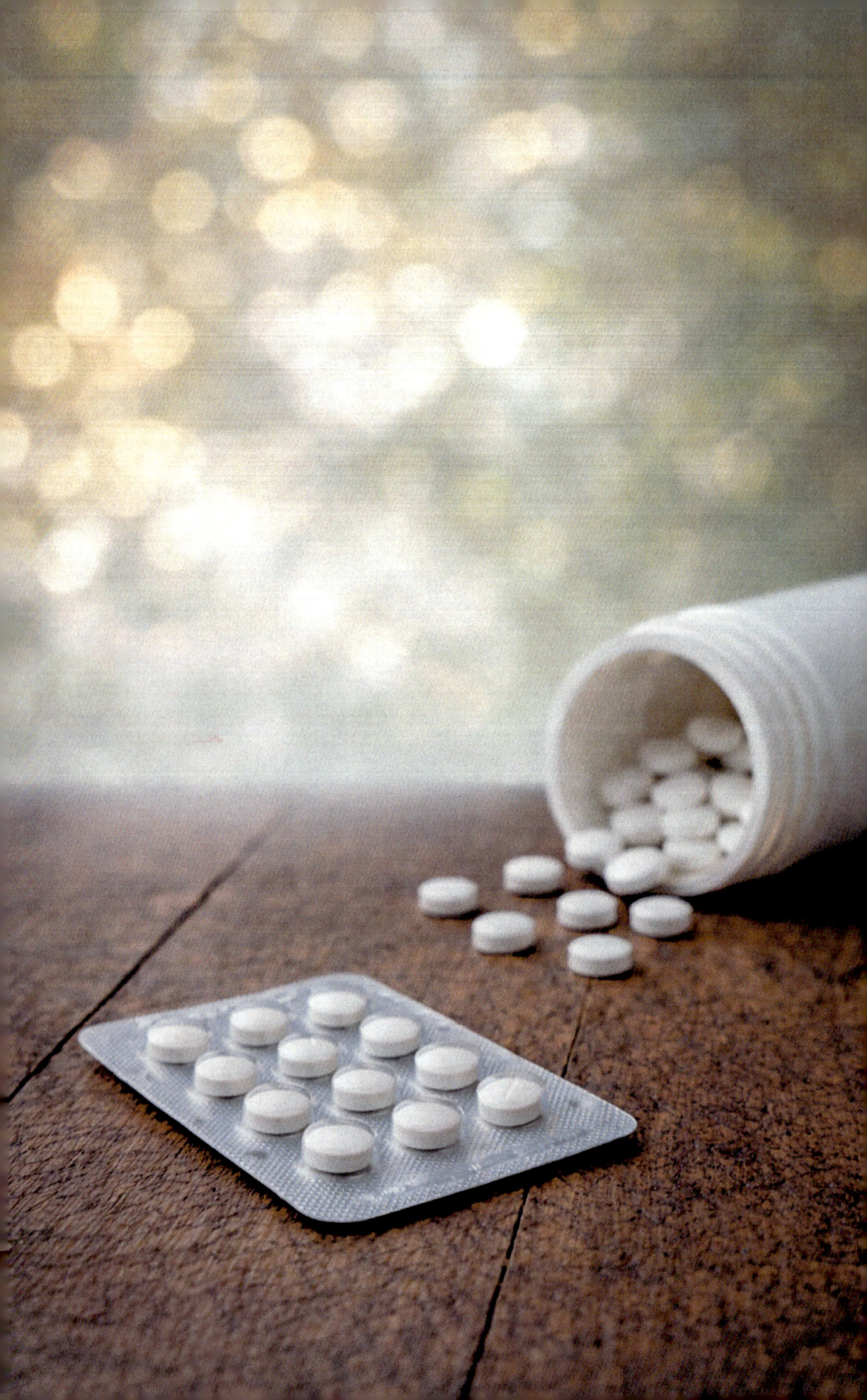

CHAPTER 8
SYNTHETIC PARASITE ELIMINATORS

THE ELEPHANT IN THE ROOM – IVERMECTIN AND FENBENDAZOLE

After working through the natural agents in the previous chapter, it helps to name an uncomfortable truth: natural is best, but it is not always enough for every case. Herbs, botanicals, binders, and rotation strategies can be remarkably effective at supporting the body's terrain and reducing unwanted organisms. Even so, there are situations where symptoms persist, the suspected load is high, or the person is too depleted to keep rotating through long protocols. In those cases, some practitioners consider a short, targeted course of a synthetic antiparasitic medication as a bridge.

This is where ivermectin comes in. In many naturopathic and holistic circles, ivermectin is discussed more than people admit, often without clear understanding of what ivermectin is, and sadly with a completely wrong understanding.

WHAT IVERMECTIN IS — AND IS NOT

Ivermectin is a synthetic antiparasitic medication used worldwide for certain parasitic infections. Its origin story begins in nature, with compounds discovered from soil organisms, then refined into a standardized pharmaceutical. That detail matters, because it helps explain why some in the natural community feel comfortable with it. Still, refined and standardized means what it means: it is synthetic. Ivermectin is not "basically natural." It is a drug. Drugs can be appropriate in the right context, and drugs can also be misused.

THE NOBEL PRIZE CONTEXT

The scientific pathway that led to ivermectin's development contributed to the 2015 Nobel Prize in Physiology or Medicine, recognizing the impact of antiparasitic discoveries on global health. This is one reason ivermectin has a certain halo around it. People hear "Nobel Prize" and assume "safe," "validated," or "universally good."

A Nobel Prize confirms significance. It does not guarantee safety for every person, every dose, or every case. It highlights that ivermectin has legitimate antiparasitic value. It does not turn it into an everyday wellness tool.

WHY HOLISTIC PRACTITIONERS SOMETIMES USE IT

Some integrative and naturopathic practitioners consider ivermectin when the situation calls for a more direct, time-bound intervention. The reasoning is usually practical: ivermectin has documented antiparasitic activity, it can act more quickly than many botanicals, and it may be used when the person has stalled after a thorough natural protocol.

The key is short term. In a holistic framework, ivermectin is best positioned as a targeted tool used within a larger plan that still prioritizes terrain, digestion, elimination, and immune function. Using a pharmaceutical does not cancel holistic principles. It simply means the practitioner judged that the risk of doing nothing or moving too slowly outweighed the risk of a monitored short course.

THE "GREENWASHING" EFFECT

The COVID era poured gasoline on this topic. Ivermectin became culturally and politically charged, and so, some natural-health communities reacted by embracing it more strongly, and sometimes too uncritically. When institutions push hard in one direction, counter-movements often push hard in the other.

In some circles, ivermectin was quietly "greenwashed" into something it is not. Claims like "it's basically natural," "it's completely safe," or "it's good for ongoing prevention" are not evidence-based. Reaction is not the same as discernment. Ivermectin is a synthetic medication that may be appropriate in limited circumstances, not a natural tonic.

THE REAL RISK: OVERUSE AND CASUAL USE

The biggest danger is that people treat it like an herb. Ivermectin is designed for short, targeted use, not continuous dosing, not constant cycling, and not long-term "prevention."

When it is overused or misused, risk climbs. Potential problems include liver stress, neurological side effects at higher exposures, drug interactions, microbiome disruption, and the false confidence that can delay proper evaluation. More is not better. Longer is not safer. Short-term tool, not lifestyle supplement.

THE HORSE PASTE PROBLEM

One of the most concerning trends has been people using veterinary ivermectin intended for horses or livestock. This is where "confidence" becomes carelessness. Even when the active ingredient is similar, veterinary products differ in concentration, dosing assumptions, fillers, and quality-control standards. Human self-dosing with animal formulations creates a real risk of overdose and adverse effects, especially when people measure by guesswork. Veterinary ivermectin is not a safe workaround. The consequences can be serious and have landed many people in the hospital due to overdosing.

SYNTHETIC EXPOSURE IN PERSPECTIVE

Some people assume if it's synthetic, then it's toxic. The truth is more nuanced. We live in a world of constant synthetic exposures in our air, water, food additives, household chemicals, personal care products, medications, and yes, synthetic isolates used in many supplements. The body is already performing heavy detox work every day.

That said, "we already have toxins" is not a permission slip to stack more. A short, medically supervised course of a medication is not the same as chronic chemical bombardment, yet synthetic is still synthetic, and the liver still has to process what we choose to bring in. Dose, duration, quality, and context matter.

HOW IVERMECTIN FITS WITHIN A PARASITE CLEANSE

When used appropriately, ivermectin is best positioned as a short intervention inside a broader framework. That framework still includes hydration, bowel regularity, and binder support when appropriate, because the goal is not only to "hit" organisms, but to clear debris and reduce recirculation. Many people tolerate short courses better when they are supporting elimination and not constipated, dehydrated, or nutritionally depleted.

GENERAL DOSING PRINCIPLE (U.S. Measurements)

For most intestinal roundworms, ivermectin is prescribed at: approximately 0.09 mg per pound of body weight. It is typically given as a single oral dose in many cases.

Example Dosing by Body Weight:

- 130 lb adult – 12 mg single dose
- 165 lb adult – 15 mg single dose
- 200 lb adult – 18 mg single dose

WHY DURATION IS OFTEN SHORT

Unlike antibiotics that target bacteria, ivermectin works by:

- Binding to glutamate-gated chloride channels in parasites
- Causing paralysis of the parasites
- Leading to death and elimination of parasites

NOTE: For many nematodes (roundworms), a single dose is sufficient because it paralyzes adult worms. Eggs may not be fully affected, which is why some protocols repeat dosing after 1–2 weeks.

RISKS WITH CHRONIC DAILY USE

Some clinicians express concern about daily long-term ivermectin use because existing safety data are based primarily on short-course treatment protocols. Chronic exposure has not been extensively studied and raises considerations related to cumulative dosing, liver metabolism, neurologic tolerance, and immune signaling effects over time.

Potential concerns:

- Liver enzyme elevation
- Drug interactions (especially those metabolized via CYP3A4)
- Neurologic effects at higher systemic levels
- Unknown long-term immune modulation

FENBENDAZOLE

Alongside ivermectin, another name that often surfaces in the same conversations is fenbendazole. It shows up in forums, podcasts, and alternative health circles, frequently mentioned alongside parasite cleansing and other off-label uses. Because of that rising visibility, it deserves the same clear and grounded treatment.

The natural approach still stands as first line: build terrain, use botanicals, support elimination, rotate wisely. Prescription medications may sometimes have a short-term role under supervision. Fenbendazole sits in a different category altogether. It is primarily a synthetic veterinary deworming drug.

WHAT FENBENDAZOLE IS — AND WHY THAT MATTERS

Fenbendazole belongs to a class of antiparasitic drugs commonly used in animals to treat intestinal worms and related organisms. It works by disrupting parasite cellular structure and energy metabolism. In veterinary medicine, it has a long track record when used at labeled doses for specific species.

What creates confusion is simple: people see that it works against parasites and assume the rest of the conclusions for themselves. Effectiveness in animals does not automatically translate into safety and appropriateness in humans. Species metabolize drugs differently. Formulations differ. Safety data differs. Fenbendazole is a veterinary medication first, not a general human wellness tool.

WHY IT HAS GAINED ATTENTION IN HOLISTIC SPACES

Interest in fenbendazole has grown largely through anecdotal reports and online communities that promote drug repurposing. Distrust of institutions plus stories of individual success can create rapid adoption before solid human evidence and safety frameworks are in place.

Some practitioners discuss it quietly. Most conventional clinicians do not recommend it for routine human use because approval, dosing standards, and large-scale safety data are limited compared with approved human medications. That tension should not be hidden. It should be named plainly. Some people group fenbendazole and ivermectin together. That is a mistake in clinical category.

Prescription human ivermectin, when used appropriately, comes with physician oversight, pharmacy quality control, and established human dosing guidelines for certain conditions. Fenbendazole typically does not.

THE REAL RISKS PEOPLE UNDERESTIMATE

Because fenbendazole is commonly used in animals, some assume it must be broadly safe. That assumption skips several important variables. Human safety data is limited compared with approved human drugs. Veterinary products may include excipients not designed for human intake. Online dosing charts are not medical guidance.

Potential concerns include liver enzyme elevation, drug interactions, formulation impurities, and dosing miscalculation. The risk increases when people stack multiple antiparasitic drugs, extend duration, or repeat cycles without lab monitoring.

The most common danger is not one dose – it's unsupervised repetition.

HARM-REDUCTION FRAMING

Harm-reduction framing gives protective clarity rather than an endorsement. If you are determined to pursue fenbendazole despite cautions, safer boundaries would include:

- Involve a licensed clinician, not forum advice
- Use pharmaceutical-grade sourcing only, not random vendors
- Check baseline and follow-up liver labs
- Avoid combining with other liver-stress agents
- Keep duration short, not open-ended
- Stop immediately if neurological or severe digestive symptoms appear

A GROUNDED CONCLUSION

Fenbendazole is not natural. Not approved as a routine human antiparasitic. Not risk-free. Not automatically wrong. Not casually safe. It is a veterinary drug that has drawn human interest faster than human evidence. Discernment means resisting both extremes: blind enthusiasm and automatic dismissal. Short-term, supervised, case-specific decisions are one thing. Internet-driven self-protocols are another. Be careful!

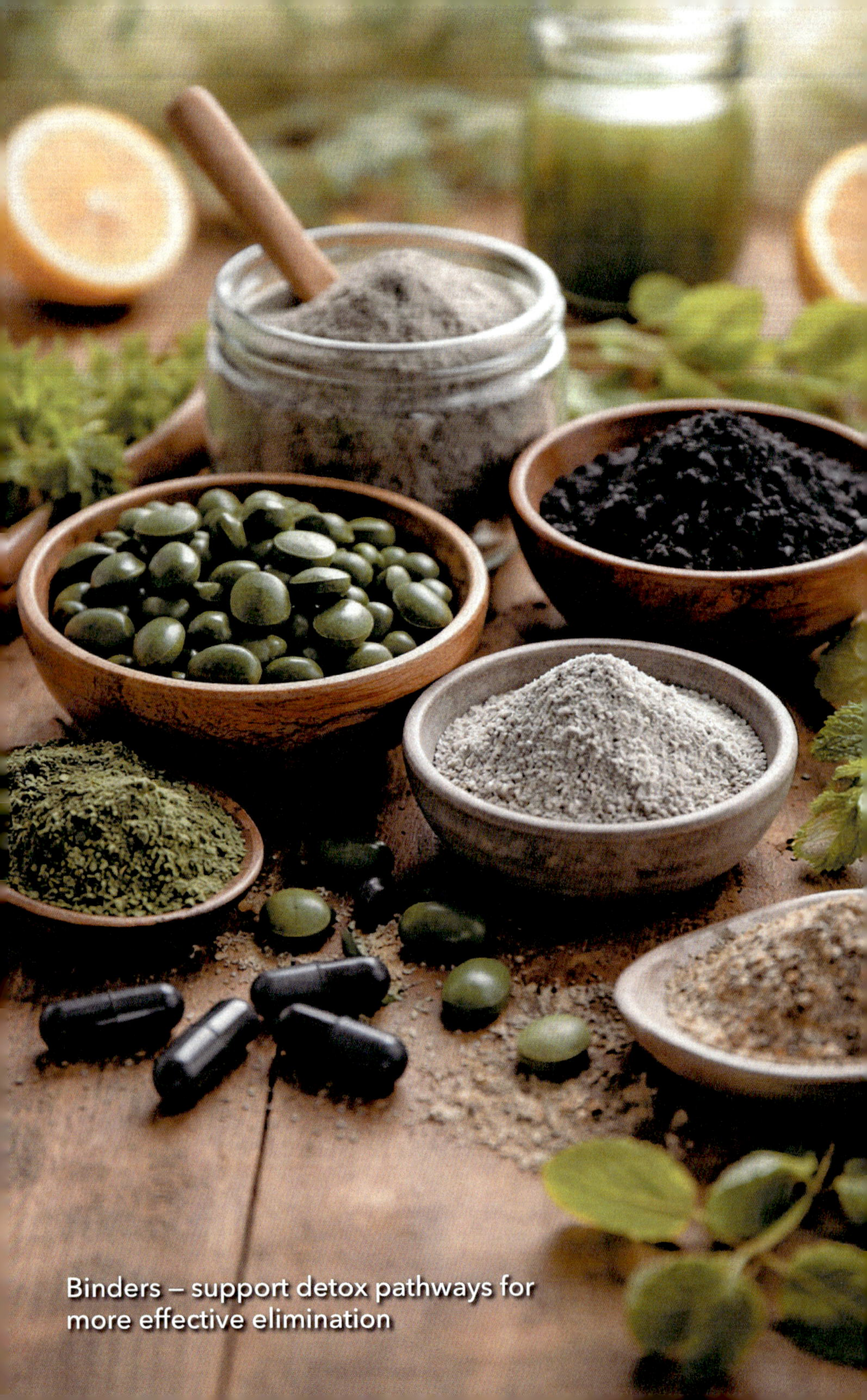

Binders – support detox pathways for more effective elimination

CHAPTER 9
BINDERS & DETOX COMPOUNDS

Parasite protocols must be about killing as well as clearing them. When organisms die, debris remains, metabolic waste circulates, and inflammatory byproducts move through lymph, liver, bile, and bowel. If those pathways are sluggish, people feel it quickly with symptoms such as headaches, fatigue, skin flare-ups, brain fog, and irritability. What was meant to help, suddenly feels overwhelming.

Sometimes these temporary symptom flares are referred to as a Herxheimer reaction, herxing, or "die-off." As organisms break down, inflammatory compounds increase temporarily. The solution is rarely stronger killing. It is usually better drainage and elimination.

This chapter supports your parasite cleanse by giving you strategic and structured binding methods to effectively remove the debris.

BINDERS AND TIMING

Binders are compounds that physically bind toxins and waste inside the gut so they can be escorted out through the stool instead of being reabsorbed. When parasites die, they release metabolic waste, endotoxins, and often stored environmental toxins. Without binding support, some of that material can recirculate through enterohepatic recycling. That recirculation is often what drives the uncomfortable "detox" symptoms people experience.

Common binders include:

- Activated charcoal
- Bentonite clay
- Chlorella
- Humic and fulvic acids (soil derived)
- Zeolite (volcanic mineral)
- Modified citrus pectin

Each binder has a slightly different affinity profile. Some are particularly helpful for endotoxins – tiny toxic pieces of certain bacteria that get released when the bacteria die and can make your body feel inflamed and achy. Others are better known for binding heavy metals. Some act more broadly. The goal is not to take them all at once, but to choose wisely and use them intentionally at specific times of day.

Timing matters more than most people realize. Binders should always be taken away from food consumption, medications, supplements, and antiparasitic herbs. If taken too close to nutrients or herbs, they will bind the helpful compounds along with the waste. A common rhythm is to take antiparasitic compounds earlier in the day and use a binder one to two hours later or at lunchtime, well away from everything else.

Hydration is important when using binders. Binders require adequate water to move effectively. Without sufficient hydration, they can slow motility, which works against the entire purpose of detoxification.

Active detoxification increases fluid and mineral turnover. With increased bowel movements and binder use, electrolytes can be depleted more quickly. Supporting sodium, potassium, magnesium, and trace minerals helps maintain energy, proper motility, and overall resilience during a cleanse.

BILE SUPPORT AND LIVER SUPPORT

The liver processes – bile carries – the bowel eliminates. If bile is thick, sluggish, or insufficient, detox slows dramatically. Parasite waste and inflammatory compounds depend on healthy bile flow for removal. Supporting bile is about encouraging steady, healthy flow and protecting liver function along the way.

Common bile and liver supports include:

- Milk thistle seed – antioxidant and hepatoprotective support
- Dandelion root – supports bile production and gentle bile flow
- Artichoke leaf – encourages bile secretion and supports fat digestion
- Beet root – supports liver detox and healthy methylation processes
- Taurine – assists with bile acid conjugation
- Glycine – assists with bile acid conjugation
- Phosphatidylcholine – supports bile integrity and cell membranes
- Bitter herbs – stimulate digestion and natural bile release

Sometimes the body gives subtle clues that bile needs attention. Pale or floating stools can indicate poor fat digestion. Fat intolerance, nausea after fatty meals, or a dull ache in the right upper quadrant may signal sluggish flow. These signs are not reasons for panic, but they are invitations to seek additional support.

The liver also requires adequate protein to function well. Detoxification pathways depend on amino acids. Undereating protein while attempting a parasite protocol often backfires. Flow requires fuel, so eat more protein during parasite cleanses.

A NOTE FOR THOSE WITHOUT A GALLBLADDER

If you have had your gallbladder removed, your body still produces bile. The liver continues to make it. What changes is storage and concentration. The gallbladder's role was to concentrate bile and release it in a strong, timed surge when fat entered the small intestine. Without it, bile drips continuously in smaller amounts rather than being released in a coordinated pulse.

This can mean less concentrated bile, reduced fat tolerance, slower clearance of fat-bound toxins, and an increased likelihood of loose stools or, conversely, sluggish digestion. During a parasite or detox protocol, this can make a difference.

Binders rely on adequate bile flow to help escort fat-soluble toxins into the intestinal tract. If bile flow is already reduced or less concentrated, toxins may not be mobilized and carried as efficiently. In some cases, people without a gallbladder may feel more sluggish during detox or may need additional bile support.

Those without a gallbladder may benefit from:

- Bitter herbs to gently stimulate bile production
- Taurine and glycine to support bile acid formation
- Phosphatidylcholine for bile consistency
- Digestive enzymes that include bile salts with higher-fat meals

At the same time, be cautious not to overload binders without ensuring motility is strong. Motility is the movement of food and waste through the digestive tract. Without a gallbladder, digestion can already be sensitive. Adequate hydration, consistent bowel movements, and moderate fat intake during active detox often make the process smoother.

Trust that your liver is still capable.
Support the flow and respect the adjustment.

MOTILITY SUPPORT

If food and waste do not move, they do not leave. This is one of the most overlooked elements in parasite protocols. Daily bowel movements are foundational. During active detoxification, one to three well-formed bowel movements per day is often ideal. When the colon is sluggish, toxins sit longer than they should: they ferment, they irritate, and they can be reabsorbed. Many people discover that when symptoms increase during a protocol, the issue is not that they need stronger antiparasitics, but that they need better motility.

Motility support may include:

- Magnesium citrate or magnesium oxide
- Vitamin C to bowel tolerance
- Aloe vera inner leaf
- Triphala
- Ginger
- Proper hydration
- Daily movement
- Individualized fiber support

A note about fiber: interestingly, fiber is highly individualized. Some people thrive when it is increased gradually. Others feel bloated and worse if it is added too quickly. The goal is not aggressive purging, but more of a consistent and complete elimination. If elimination slows, adjust first before escalating intensity. Clear pathways so you calm reactions.

LYMPHATIC SUPPORT

The lymphatic system helps transport cellular waste and inflammatory byproducts out of tissues. Unlike the cardiovascular system, it does not have a central pump. It depends on movement and muscle contraction. When lymph becomes stagnant, detox can feel heavier. Swelling, puffiness, fatigue, and sluggish recovery may increase.

Lymphatic support may include:

- Rebounding or gentle bouncing like jumping jacks
- Walking
- Dry brushing
- Adequate hydration
- Deep diaphragmatic breathing

Movement is medicine for lymph. Always remember that gentle consistency is more effective than higher intensity.

NERVOUS SYSTEM REGULATION

Detoxification is biochemical and also neurological. The body eliminates most efficiently in a parasympathetic state. This is the "rest and digest" mode governed by the vagus nerve.

When the nervous system is chronically stressed, bile flow slows, motility becomes irregular, and inflammation increases. A cleanse layered on top of stress can amplify symptoms.

Nervous system support may include:

- Adequate sleep
- Unhurried meals
- Deep breathing
- Time outdoors
- Gentle movement rather than overtraining

Remember: calm physiology clears more efficiently than a stressed one.

GUT-SOOTHING SUPPORTS

Parasites irritate the intestinal lining. Strong herbs can be drying or inflammatory when used aggressively. Even when necessary, they can create collateral irritation if the terrain is not supported.

The intestinal lining is not simply a tube. It is a barrier, an immune interface, and a communication hub. Supporting its integrity helps maintain healthy immune function and reduces inflammation.

Soothing and reparative compounds may include:

- Slippery elm
- Marshmallow root
- L-glutamine
- Zinc L-carnosine
- Deglycyrrhizinated licorice
- Collagen
- Bone broth
- Aloe vera inner leaf

These compounds support mucosal integrity, calm irritation, and assist epithelial repair. When layered into a protocol thoughtfully, they allow the body to address parasites without unnecessarily compromising the overall health of your terrain.

PUTTING IT ALL TOGETHER

A structured parasite protocol is rhythmic and intentional. Antiparasitic compounds are used with purpose. Binders are layered in strategically. Liver and bile support should be maintained daily. Motility is monitored consistently and gut support is not an afterthought.

It is important to remember that symptoms are information. If reactions escalate, do not automatically intensify the protocol. Often the solution is improved drainage, not stronger killing. Trust the process. When elimination functions well, healing becomes steadier, smoother, and far more sustainable.

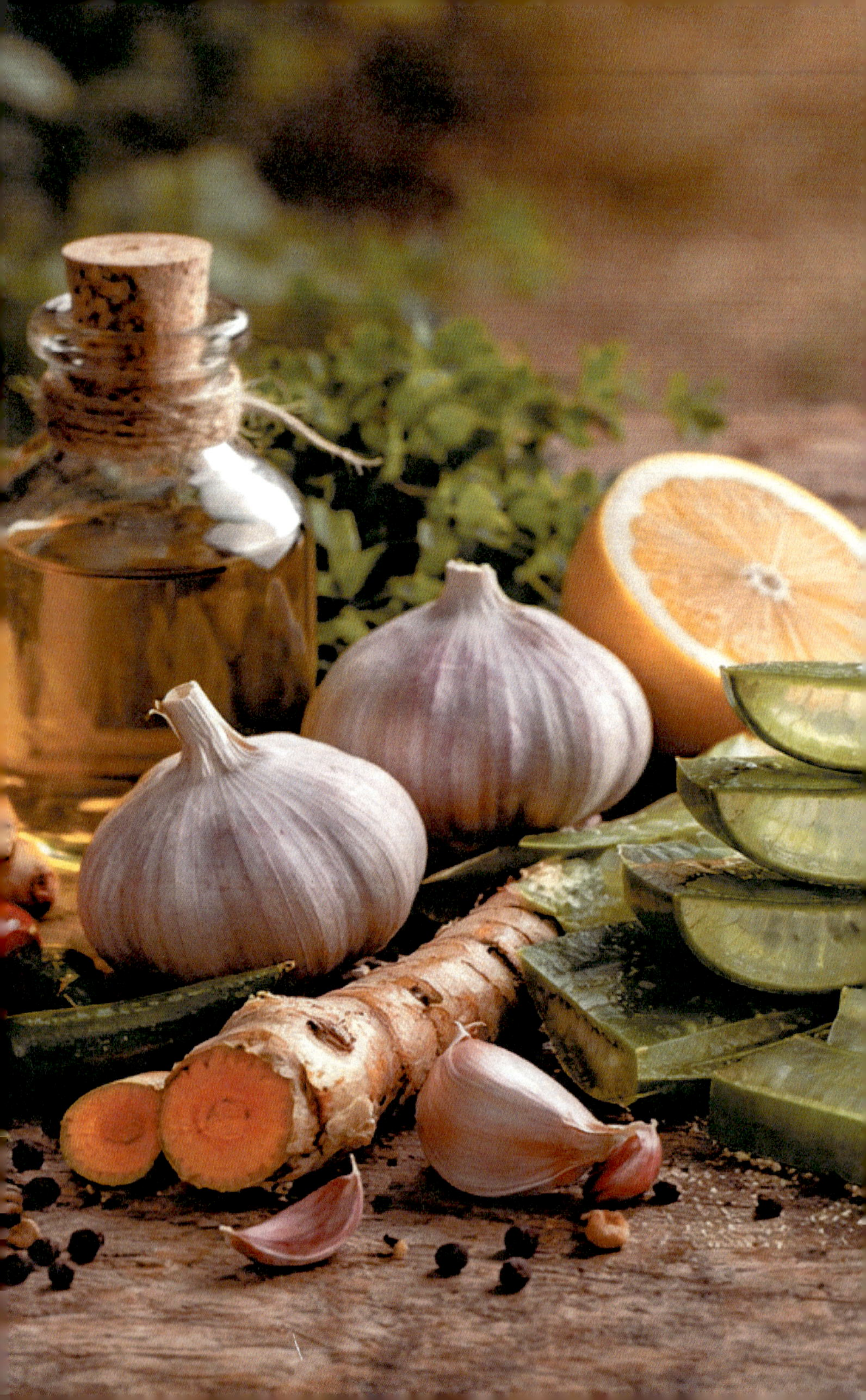

PART TWO

PARASITE PROTOCOL

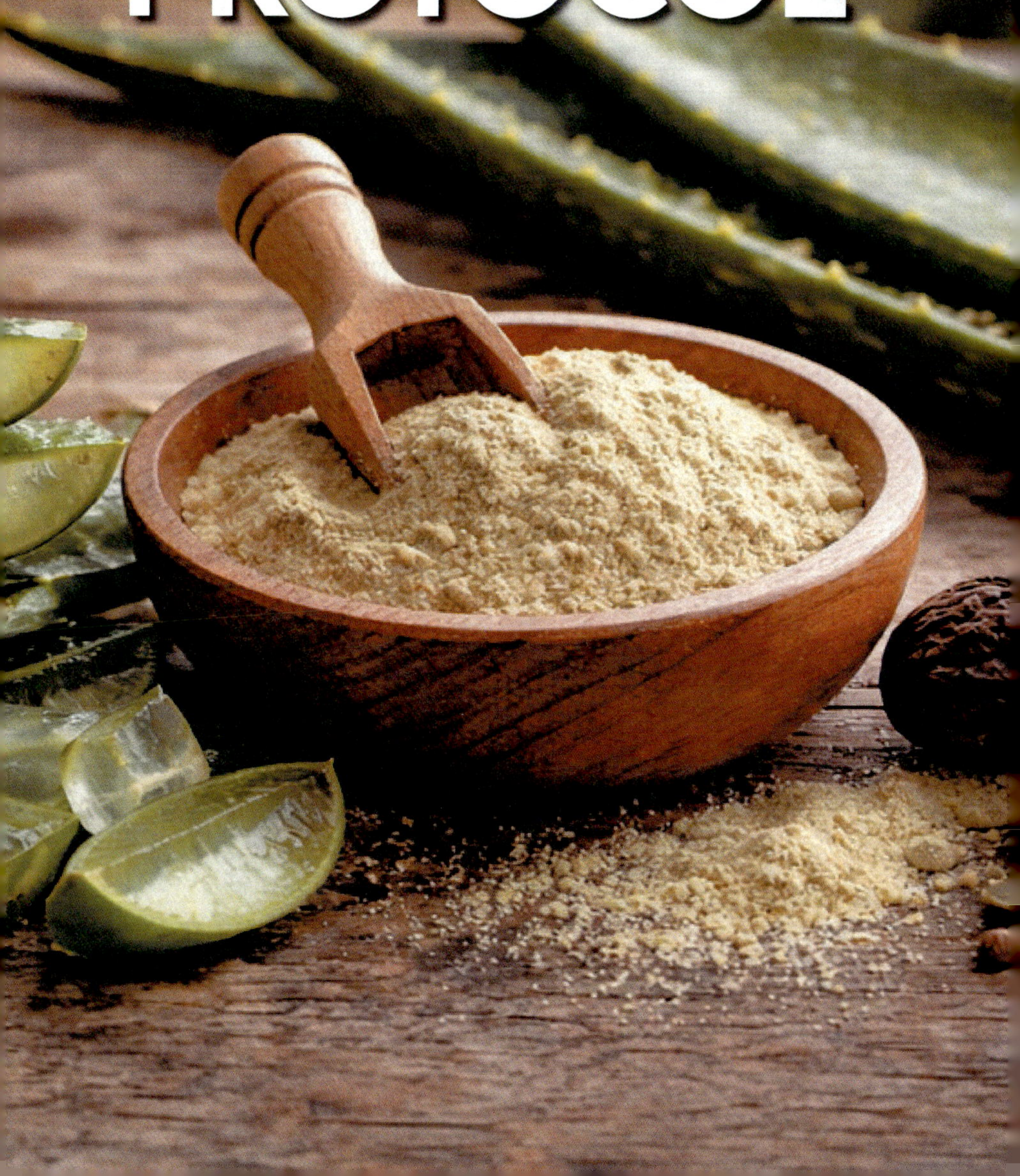

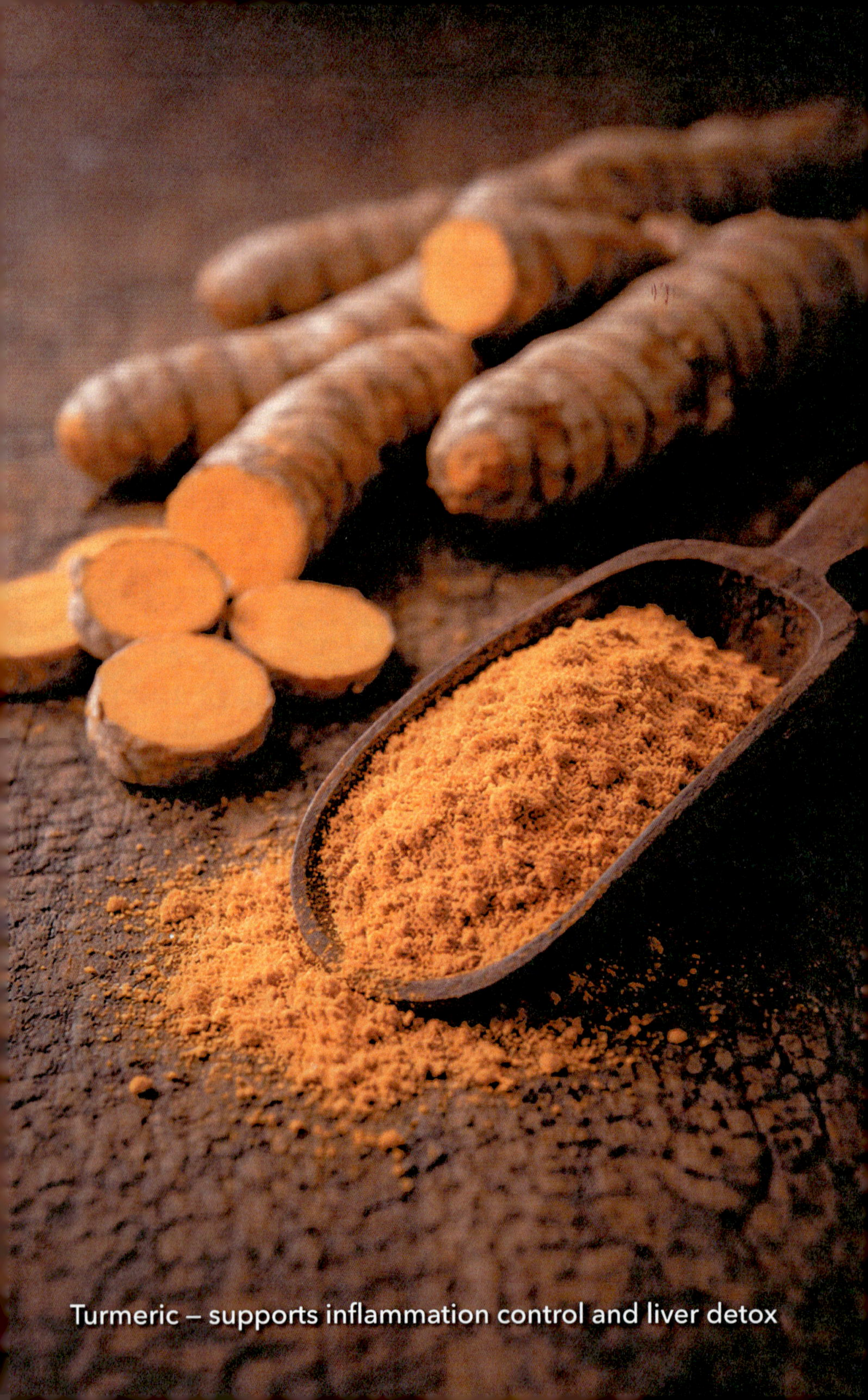

Turmeric – supports inflammation control and liver detox

CHAPTER 10
PREPARATION

PREPARATION PHASE

Before beginning any parasite protocol, it is important to pause and assess readiness. Detoxification is not something to rush into simply because it is trending or because someone else reported dramatic results. The body functions through order and design. When we respect that design, outcomes are far more stable and sustainable.

Parasite cleansing places stress on detoxification pathways. Even when done gently, it mobilizes waste, inflammatory debris, and stored compounds that must be properly processed and eliminated. If elimination pathways are sluggish or nutritional reserves are low, symptoms can intensify unnecessarily. Preparation is a very important part of the protocol.

"Plans succeed with many counselors." – Proverbs 20:18 (NKJV)
Wise preparation protects the individual from avoidable setbacks.

THE HEAVY METAL DEBATE

One of the most common questions in parasite work is whether heavy metals must be addressed first. Some practitioners argue that metals should always be detoxified before parasites. Their reasoning is that parasites can accumulate heavy metals, and killing parasites may release those metals back into circulation.

There is some biological plausibility to this idea. Certain organisms and biofilms can bind environmental toxins, including metals such as mercury, lead, and cadmium. However, the conclusion that aggressive chelation must precede parasite cleansing does not apply universally.

Chelation therapy mobilizes stored metals from tissues. Once mobilized, those metals must be eliminated effectively through the liver, bile, kidneys, and bowels. If bowel movements are irregular, hydration is inadequate, or mineral status is compromised, redistribution can occur and symptoms may worsen.

Another important factor is mineral balance. Heavy metals often displace essential minerals such as magnesium, zinc, selenium, and other trace elements. If someone is already depleted, mobilizing metals without first restoring mineral sufficiency can create additional instability. For most people, a more prudent approach is to prioritize stabilization before aggressive metal detoxification.

Stabilization includes ensuring:

- Regular bowel movements
- Adequate hydration
- Sufficient protein intake
- Repletion of essential minerals
- Gentle support of liver and lymphatic function

When the body is nourished and elimination pathways are functioning well, it is better equipped to handle both parasitic debris and environmental toxin burden in a measured way.

There are, of course, exceptions. Documented heavy metal toxicity, significant occupational exposure, or recent improper amalgam filling removal may warrant targeted metal support under professional supervision. Even in those cases, foundational stabilization is essential.

An overburden of heavy metals is not insignificant. Yet in parasite cleansing, the question is not whether metals matter, but when to address them. In most cases, the body responds best when foundational systems are strengthened and supported first, followed by a measured approach to deeper burdens such as heavy metals.

READINESS CHECKLIST

Before beginning a parasite protocol, the following should be in place:

Bowel Function – Daily elimination is essential. If bowel movements are inconsistent or infrequent, toxins released during parasite die-off can be reabsorbed. Chronic constipation should be addressed before beginning any cleansing protocol.

Hydration – Adequate hydration supports lymphatic circulation, kidney function, and bile flow. Urine should generally be light in color. Electrolyte and mineral support may be appropriate, especially for individuals prone to depletion.

Mineral Status – Mineral sufficiency supports immune function and detoxification pathways. Particular attention should be given to magnesium, zinc, selenium, and trace minerals. Restoration should precede aggressive detoxification.

Protein Intake – The liver requires amino acids for Phase I and Phase II detoxification processes. Individuals who are undereating, fasting aggressively, or consuming insufficient protein should correct this before beginning a parasite cleanse. Preparation ensures that when mobilization occurs, elimination can keep pace.

SETTING EXPECTATIONS

Parasite protocols are rarely dramatic when implemented thoughtfully. Some individuals notice minimal changes. Others experience temporary fatigue, mild digestive shifts, or transient discomfort as the body adjusts. More intense reactions do not necessarily indicate greater effectiveness. In fact, excessive die-off can signal that the protocol is too aggressive for the current state of the body. The goal is steady progress, not intensity. Improvement is often gradual and measured over weeks, or even months, rather than days.

BASELINE TRACKING

Before starting, it is helpful to document current symptoms and patterns. This provides a reference point for evaluating progress and prevents over-interpretation of normal fluctuations.

Consider recording:

- Energy levels
- Sleep quality
- Bowel frequency and consistency
- Skin changes
- Lessening joint discomfort
- Mental clarity
- Food cravings
- Mood stability

WHEN NOT TO START

There are situations in which a parasite detox should be postponed.

These include:

- Pregnancy or breastfeeding
- Severe constipation
- Acute illness or infection
- Post-surgical recovery
- Significant adrenal exhaustion
- Periods of extreme emotional or physiological stress
- Active eating disorders or severe caloric restriction

NOTE: A parasite detox may be initiated at any time of year when elimination pathways are open, hydration is consistent, and foundational nutrition is stable. Some traditions suggest beginning on a full moon due to the belief that certain parasites are more active during lunar brightness, possibly linked to historical observations of nocturnal behavior and gravitational rhythms. Modern physiology does not require lunar timing for effectiveness. Structured sequencing, proper preparation, and steady support determine outcomes far more than the phase of the moon.

WEEK 1 – PREPARATION

Before introducing antimicrobial herbs or rotating binders, the body must demonstrate that elimination pathways are functioning and nutritional reserves are adequate. Week 1 strengthens the terrain so that when mobilization begins, the body can process what is released.

Primary Goals of Week 1

- Establish consistent daily bowel movements
- Improve hydration and mineral intake
- Ensure adequate protein consumption
- Begin gentle liver and lymphatic support
- Assess tolerance to mild binders

Nothing in this week should feel aggressive. If symptoms worsen during Week 1, that is useful information. It indicates the body needs further stabilization before proceeding.

DAILY FOUNDATIONS

1. Bowel Regularity

The goal is at least one comfortable bowel movement daily. If bowel movements are inconsistent, begin with gentle strategies:

- Increase water intake
- Add magnesium as tolerated
- Increase dietary fiber gradually
- Include cooked vegetables and healthy fats
- Add light movement such as walking

If constipation persists, delay Phase 1. Mobilizing toxins without elimination is counterproductive.

2. Hydration and Minerals

Aim for steady hydration throughout the day rather than large amounts at once. Mineralized fluids are often preferable to plain water for individuals who are depleted. Support may include:

- Trace mineral drops
- Magnesium
- Potassium-rich whole foods
- Broths

Hydration supports lymphatic flow and bile movement. Without it, detoxification slows.

3. Protein Sufficiency
Detoxification requires amino acids. During Week 1, ensure adequate protein intake daily. Most individuals benefit from approximately 0.7–1 gram of protein per pound of ideal body weight, adjusted for individual needs and tolerance. Undereating during detox increases fatigue and slows repair. Protein sources should be clean, well-tolerated, and distributed evenly throughout the day.

4. Gentle Liver and Lymphatic Support
This is not the week for aggressive liver flushing. Instead, support the body's natural processes. Daily practices may include:

- Bitters before meals
- Light movement
- Dry brushing
- Deep breathing
- Adequate sleep

These practices improve circulation and drainage without overwhelming the system.

5. Binder Assessment
Before beginning antimicrobial herbs, it is wise to test tolerance to a gentle binder in small amounts. Start slow and observe for:

- Constipation
- Headache
- Increased fatigue
- Significant digestive discomfort

If strong reactions occur even at low doses, further preparation may be needed. Sometimes the body requires more mineral support or improved bowel regularity before tolerating binders.

WHAT YOU SHOULD NOTICE BY THE END OF WEEK 1

By the end of Week 1, most individuals should experience:

- More consistent bowel movements
- Improved hydration status
- Slightly more stable energy
- Fewer cravings
- Greater awareness of baseline symptoms

If symptoms are unstable or worsening, extend Week 1 rather than progressing to Phase 1. There is no prize for moving quickly. Once elimination is consistent, hydration is adequate, protein intake is stable, and mild binders are tolerated, you are ready to begin Phase 1.

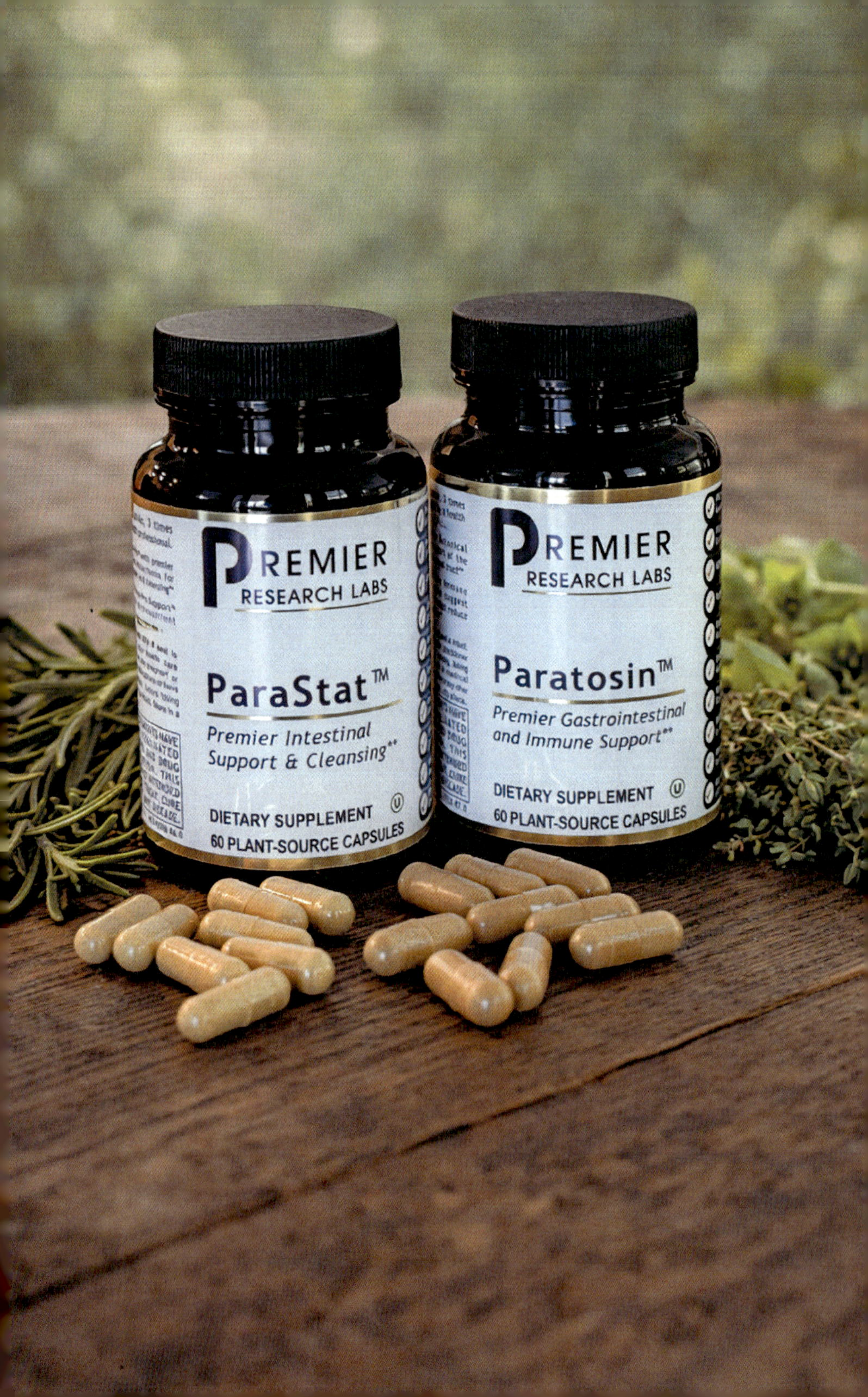
PREMIER
RESEARCH LABS
ParaStat™
Premier Intestinal Support & Cleansing**
DIETARY SUPPLEMENT
60 PLANT-SOURCE CAPSULES
PREMIER
RESEARCH LABS
Paratosin™
Premier Gastrointestinal and Immune Support**
DIETARY SUPPLEMENT
60 PLANT-SOURCE CAPSULES

CHAPTER 11

PARASITE DETOX SUPPLEMENTS

OPTIONAL SHOPPING LIST:

Fullscript: https://us.fullscript.com/plans/josullivan-holistic-parasite-detox

Essential for Detox (or find alternative with similar ingredients):

- 1 bottle Gaia Herbs Microbiome Cleanse
- 1 bottle Gaia Herbs Wormwood Black Walnut Supreme
- 2 bottles PRL ParaStat
- 2 bottles PRL Paratosin (often only from PRL)

Suggested Support for Detox:

- 3 bottles PRL BiliVen
- 2 bottles PRL Microbiome-18
- 1 bottle PRL Premier Probiotic (60 caps)
- 2 bottles PRL Medi-Chlorella-FX or Codeage Full Spectrum Binder+
- 2 bottles PRL Premier Aloe or Global Healing Aloe Vera
- 2 bottles Turmeric such as PRL Premier Turmeric (optional)
- 2 bottles Digestive Enzyme such as PRL Premier Digest (optional)

Note: For a discount on your Premier Research Labs (PRL) supplements, please text PRL to 949-868-0313.

HERBAL SUPPLEMENTS

Gaia Herbs Microbiome Cleanse – Foundational antimicrobial. Gaia Herbs Microbiome Cleanse provides broad botanical support for digestive balance and microbial regulation. In this protocol, it serves as the early-phase primer, introducing controlled microbial pressure in Phase 1 and preparing the terrain for more targeted strategies in Phase 2.

Gaia Herbs Wormwood Black Walnut Supreme – Targeted antimicrobial escalation. This formula provides concentrated herbal support for intestinal cleansing, using wormwood and black walnut hull to apply direct antimicrobial pressure. In this protocol, it serves as a Phase 2 escalation once elimination pathways are stable.

ParaStat – Primary botanical antimicrobial support. ParaStat provides broad-spectrum herbal pressure against parasites and unwanted microbial overgrowth. It works by creating an inhospitable terrain for organisms while supporting the body's natural immune response. In this protocol, it is one half of the active antimicrobial strategy during ON weeks.

Paratosin – Targeted parasite-focused botanical support. Paratosin complements ParaStat by adding deeper, more specific pressure against parasitic organisms. Used together, they create layered antimicrobial activity without relying on synthetic medication. Cycling prevents overstimulation and protects the microbiome.

BiliVen – Bile flow and liver support. Bile is essential for detoxification. Bile is essential for toxin clearance through stool. BiliVen supports healthy bile production and flow during die-off phases, helping reduce stagnation and recirculation. It is used during ON and OFF weeks and is especially helpful for those without a gallbladder.

Microbiome-18 – Terrain and microbiome support. Microbiome-18 helps maintain microbial balance during antimicrobial use. While ParaStat and Paratosin apply pressure, Microbiome-18 supports competitive exclusion and overall gut ecosystem stability. It helps reduce rebound overgrowth during OFF weeks.

Medi-Chlorella-FX – Binds toxins and wastes to lessen detox symptoms. Chlorella binds toxins released during microbial die-off so they can be eliminated through the stool rather than reabsorbed. Proper spacing is critical. In this protocol, it reduces Herxheimer reactions and protects gut integrity during ON weeks, with continued light use during OFF weeks.

Codeage Full Spectrum Binder+ – Comprehensive toxin binding. This formula combines multiple binders to help capture microbial debris and metabolic waste during a parasite detox, supporting efficient elimination during active phases.

Aloe – Supports the lining of the gut. Antimicrobial protocols can irritate the gut lining in sensitive individuals. Premier Aloe provides soothing support to maintain intestinal integrity and calm inflammation. It supports repair while detoxification is underway.

Turmeric – Reduces inflammation and supports the liver. Turmeric helps moderate inflammatory signaling during die-off and supports liver detox pathways. It is not a binder and not antimicrobial pressure. It is protective support, especially useful in Phases 2 and 3 when detox intensity increases.

Digestive Enzymes – Improve digestion. Digestive enzymes help break down proteins, fats, and carbohydrates, supporting nutrient absorption and reducing residue in the gut during a parasite detox. They are not binders or primary antimicrobials. They provide foundational digestive support as antimicrobial intensity increases.

INGREDIENTS & FUNCTION

Gaia Herbs Microbiome Cleanse

Gaia Microbiome Cleanse provides comprehensive botanical support for intestinal microbial balance. It combines traditional antiparasitic herbs with broad microbial modulators and digestive supports. The formula works by discouraging unwanted organisms, supporting immune vigilance, and promoting a balanced intestinal terrain.

Core Antimicrobial & Microbial Modulation Blend

Black Walnut (green hulls) extract *(Juglans nigra)*
Green black walnut hulls are a traditional herb used in parasite cleanses. They contribute botanical compounds that discourage unwanted organisms while supporting normal digestive function.

Organic Sweet Wormwood (aerial parts) *(Artemisia annua)*
Sweet wormwood is used to promote microbial balance in the gastrointestinal tract. It supports the body's natural defenses.

Organic Oregano (leaf) *(Origanum vulgare)*
Oregano leaf contains naturally occurring aromatic compounds that support healthy microbial balance with antioxidant support.

Oregon Grape (root) *(Mahonia aquifolium)*
Rich in plant alkaloids traditionally used to support gut and immune function, Oregon grape helps maintain healthy microbial equilibrium.

Andrographis (leaf) extract *(Andrographis paniculata)*
Andrographis supports immune responsiveness and helps modulate inflammatory signaling. In cleansing protocols, it contributes to balanced immune activity during microbial shifts.

Digestive Comfort & Terrain Support

Organic Cinnamon (bark) CO_2 extract *(Cinnamomum verum)*
Cinnamon bark supports healthy digestion and contributes additional botanical support for microbial balance.

Organic Peppermint (leaf) essential oil *(Mentha piperita)*
Peppermint essential oil promotes digestive comfort, supports motility, and helps ease occasional bloating or cramping.

What Gaia Herbs Microbiome Cleanse Does in the Parasite Detox

In this protocol, Gaia Microbiome Cleanse serves as the foundational botanical primer in Phase 1. It gently introduces antimicrobial pressure while supporting digestive comfort and immune balance. Its role is to begin shifting the intestinal terrain before more concentrated antimicrobial strategies are layered in later phases.

Gaia Herbs Wormwood Black Walnut Supreme
A traditional botanical blend used in parasite cleanses to help create an intestinal environment that is less favorable to unwanted organisms. It combines targeted herbs that support digestive secretions, microbial balance, and overall gut terrain during antimicrobial phases.

Active Ingredients: Black Walnut Green Hulls Extract, Sweet Wormwood, Pomegranate, Coptis Root, Gentian Root, Clove Flower Bud, and Ginger Root.

Black Walnut Green Hulls Extract
Contains tannins and juglone, which create an environment in the intestinal tract that is unfavorable to many parasites.

Organic Sweet Wormwood *(Artemisia annua)*
A bitter herb that creates oxidative stress within certain parasites, weakening or killing them, particularly protozoa.

Pomegranate (freeze-dried arils)
Provides additional phytonutrients with antioxidant properties to support overall digestive resilience.

Coptis (root) *(Coptis chinensis)*
Contains high levels of berberine, an isoquinoline alkaloid with documented antimicrobial activity.

Gentian (root) *(Gentiana lutea)*
Bitter root that supports healthy digestion by stimulating digestive secretions and promoting gentle gastrointestinal function.

Clove (bud) *(Syzygium aromaticum)*
Contains eugenol, which may help disrupt and damage parasite eggs by penetrating and destabilizing their protective outer shells, supporting life-cycle coverage during a cleanse.

Ginger (root) *(Zingiber officinale)*
Supports gastrointestinal motility and comfort.

What Gaia Herbs Wormwood Black Walnut Supreme Does in the Parasite Detox Protocol
In a parasite detox protocol, this herbal blend supports digestive terrain and helps maintain a balanced intestinal environment during antimicrobial phases. The bitter botanicals promote digestive secretions, support bile flow, and help the body stay comfortable as microbial shifts occur. It is typically used short term, taken between meals, and separated from food and other supplements to optimize effectiveness.

ParaStat

ParaStat provides broad-spectrum herbal assault against parasites and unwanted microbial overgrowth. It works by creating an inhospitable environment for organisms while supporting the immune response.

Para-Pro™ Core Blend

Holarrhena (bark) *(Holarrhena antidysenterica)*
This is the primary botanical in ParaStat. Traditionally used to support intestinal health, it helps promote a balanced gut environment and assists in clearing unwanted microbes.

Para-Pro Support™ Blend

Organic Turmeric (rhizome) *(Curcuma longa)*
A well-researched botanical that helps modulate inflammatory signaling and supports normal liver detox pathways.

Organic Hyssop (aerial parts) *(Hyssopus officinalis)*
Traditionally used to support respiratory and digestive tract comfort, hyssop adds gentle support for microbial balance.

Organic Olive (leaf) *(Olea europaea)*
Olive contains phytonutrients like oleuropein that support normal immune function, provide antioxidant support, and terrain balance.

Organic Burdock (root) *(Arctium lappa)*
A traditional herbal detoxifier, burdock root supports lymphatic and digestive systems, helping promote healthy bowel movements.

Aquamin® F Mineralized Red Algae (whole) *(Lithothamnion sp.)*
A natural source of bioavailable minerals (including calcium and magnesium) that supports intestinal environment integrity and overall mineral balance while detoxification is underway.

Organic Fennel (seed) *(Foeniculum vulgare)*
Fennel seed traditionally supports digestion, helps ease gas or bloating, and encourages smooth motility of the gastrointestinal tract.

Other Ingredients

Plant-Source Capsule (cellulose, water) — Provides vegan/vegetarian capsule delivery without animal gelatin or excipients.

What ParaStat Does in the Parasite Detox

ParaStat helps create an intestinal environment that discourages unwanted microbes while supporting smooth, natural elimination. It promotes digestive comfort by easing gas and bloating and provides botanical support to keep immune and detox pathways functioning well during antimicrobial phases.

Paratosin

Paratosin is a comprehensive botanical blend designed to support the entire gastrointestinal tract, encourage healthy immune response, and help reduce biofilm adhesion in the gut.

ParaClude™ Blend

This is the proprietary botanical blend that makes Paratosin effective.

Organic Clove (bud) *(Syzygium aromaticum)*
Supports a normal microbial environment in the digestive tract and provides antioxidant support. Traditionally used to help promote gastrointestinal comfort and balance.

Reishi (fruiting body) *(Ganoderma lucidum)*
A medicinal mushroom that supports healthy immune function and helps the body adapt to stress; also supports a balanced gut flora.

Wild Bear Garlic (leaf) *(Allium ursinum)*
Botanical ally traditionally used for digestive comfort and microbial terrain support, helping maintain present microbial balance without disrupting healthy flora.

Organic Hyssop (aerial parts) *(Hyssopus officinalis)*
Supports digestive tract comfort and may help with occasional indigestion; adds mild botanical support to microbial balance.

Aquamin® F Mineralized Red Algae (whole) *(Lithothamnion sp.)*
Provides marine-derived minerals that help support the intestinal environment and overall nutrient mineral balance during detox.

Organic Olive (leaf) *(Olea europaea)*
Contains phytonutrients such as oleuropein that support normal immune response and contribute antioxidant activity in the gut.

Other Ingredients:
Plant-source capsule (organic pullulan, water, seaweed extract) — clean delivery system without fillers.

How Paratosin Works in the Parasite Detox Protocol

This formula supports gastrointestinal balance by helping maintain a comfortable digestive environment while antimicrobial pressure is applied. It assists a healthy immune response through botanicals such as reishi and olive leaf, which provide added support as the terrain shifts. It also helps reduce biofilm adhesion by targeting microbial communication, making antimicrobial transitions more effective. At the same time, herbs like wild bear garlic, hyssop, and clove help soothe the digestive tract and ease occasional irritation during detox phases.

BiliVen

BiliVen is a gallbladder and liver support formula designed to help promote healthy bile production and flow to support detoxification even if you have had your gallbladder removed.

Vitamin B6 (as pyridoxal-5-phosphate)
A bioactive form of B6 that supports liver enzyme activity involved in detox pathways and helps metabolize fats and amino acids for bile flow.

Artichoke (leaf) Extract *(Cynara scolymus)*
Artichoke encourages healthy liver function and stimulates bile flow, helping fats break down more efficiently and promoting smoother elimination of mobilized toxins.

Organic Turmeric (rhizome) & Turmeric Extract *(Curcuma longa)*
Turmeric provides antioxidant and anti-inflammatory support to help calm inflammatory signaling and support liver detox pathways, adding an extra layer of protection during microbial die-off.

Organic Milk Thistle (seed) *(Silybum marianum)*
A classic liver herb rich in silymarin, which supports liver cell integrity and assists the liver in processing and eliminating toxins. This enhances the organ's ability to handle increased detoxification.

Organic Burdock (root) *(Arctium lappa)*
Traditionally used for cleansing support; burdock aids lymphatic flow and overall detox balance while also providing digestive comfort.

Organic Fennel (seed) *(Foeniculum vulgare)*
Supports gentle digestive ease, reducing occasional gas or bloating while promoting smooth gastrointestinal motility.

Garlic (bulb) Extract *(Allium sativum)*
Offers antioxidant compounds and supports healthy microbial balance in the gut, complementing other detox support botanicals.

Organic Beet (root) *(Beta vulgaris)*
Supports liver enzyme activity and helps during elimination phases by supporting blood flow and nutrient delivery to detox organs.

How BiliVen Supports the Parasite Detox Protocol

BiliVen supports healthy bile flow with artichoke, turmeric, and milk thistle to aid toxin mobilization and elimination. It strengthens liver function and antioxidant protection while promoting digestive comfort during detox. It also helps support bile metabolism for those without a gallbladder.

MicroBiome-18

A full-spectrum probiotic formula designed to help support healthy gut flora balance, microbial terrain recovery, and intestinal health.

Live-Source Probiotic Complex (10 billion CFU)
A blend of 16 beneficial bacterial strains, including *Lactobacillus, Bifidobacterium, Lactococcus lactis,* and *Streptococcus thermophilus*

These "good" bacteria help:

- Support a balanced microbiome, which competes with undesirable organisms during and after antimicrobial pressure
- Promote healthy digestion and nutrient breakdown
- Support normal gut immune cell signaling
- Help maintain regular elimination and reduce digestive discomfort

Each strain contributes slightly different functions (e.g., *L. rhamnosus* helps mucosal balance, *B. longum* supports butyrate production, etc.), together creating diverse terrain support.

DE111® *Bacillus subtilis* (5 billion CFU)

- A patented, hardy probiotic strain included for its unique resilience
- Survives stomach acid and reaches the intestines effectively
- Can colonize, increase its numbers, and even resporulate, helping long-term balance
- Supports immune function and crowding-out of bad microbes
- Complements the other strains by acting in areas where traditional probiotics sometimes struggle
- DE111® is one of the most clinically studied probiotic strains and was chosen for its stability and efficacy

Other Ingredients:

Rice Hull, Rice Bran, Tapioca Dextrin – Help deliver the probiotic organisms and provide prebiotic-type food to nourish them
Plant-derived capsule (hypromellose, water, gellan gum) – A clean vegetarian capsule ensures wider acceptability

What MicroBiome-18 Does in the Parasite Detox Protocol

- Repopulates beneficial bacteria after herb-driven microbial shifts
- Supports immune function during microbial turnover
- Reduces bloating by supporting digestion and motility
- Maintains microbial diversity, preventing rebound dysbiosis
- Assists terrain resilience: each detox round feels more manageable

Premier Probiotic

Premier Probiotic is a comprehensive fermented multi-culture formula designed to help restore and stabilize the intestinal microbiome during and after antimicrobial phases.

Active Ingredients:

Prebiotic Fermented Multi-Culture – 840 mg
Fermented fruits, vegetables, mushrooms, and seaweeds that act as both nutrient sources and natural prebiotic substrates.

Fruits: Prunes *(Prunus domestica)*, Goji berries *(Lycium chinense)*, Figs *(Ficus carica)*, Blueberries *(Vaccinium spp.)*, Red Bayberries *(Myrica rubra)*, Yuzu *(Citrus junos)* – These provide natural fibers, polyphenols, and phytonutrients that nourish beneficial bacteria

Vegetables (leaves and stalks): Japanese Mugwort *(Artemisia princeps)*, Komatsuna *(Brassica rapa var. perviridis)* – These contribute additional plant compounds that support gut terrain

Mushrooms (fruiting bodies): Shiitake *(Lentinula edodes)*, Agaricus *(A. blazei)*, Maitake *(Grifola frondosa)* – Medicinal mushrooms support immune and microbial equilibrium within the digestive tract

Seaweeds (leaves and stalks): Hijiki *(Hizikia fusiforme)*, Wakame *(Undaria pinnatifida)*, Kombu kelp *(Laminaria japonica)* – Provide trace minerals and polysaccharides that nourish beneficial microbes

Probiotics: from the above fermented fruits
Probiotics (50,000 CFU/g) – A multi-strain bacteria blend designed to reinforce microbial balance:

Bifidobacteria: *B. breve M-16v, B. infantis M-63, B. longum BB536*

Lactobacilli: *L. acidophilus ATCC SD5212, L. brevis NBRC 3345, L. bulgaricus NBRC 13953, L. casei TO-A, L. fermentum NBRC 3071, L. helveticus ss. jugurti BBRC 3809, L. plantarum TO-A*

Other supportive strains: *Enterococcus faecalis TH10, Streptococcus thermophilus NBRC 13597, Bacillus coagulans*

Postbiotics: includes short-chain fatty acids and other organic acids such as acetic, citric, fulvic, humic, and phenyllactic acids, along with oligosaccharides, polyphenols, and melanoidin. These help nourish colon cells, support gut lining integrity, and enhance microbial balance.

How Premier Probiotic Supports the Parasite Detox Protocol
Premier Probiotic serves as the restorative microbiome anchor during OFF weeks and after antimicrobial phases. It helps rebuild beneficial flora, stabilize the intestinal terrain, and support immune recalibration, reinforcing digestive resilience and reducing rebound overgrowth.

Medi-Chlorella-FX

A single-ingredient formula containing broken cell wall chlorella, a freshwater green microalgae. There are no herbal blends, no fillers, and no stimulants. Its effectiveness comes from the structure of the algae itself.

Active Ingredient: Broken Cell Wall Chlorella *(Chlorella pyrenoidosa)* A mechanically cracked microalgae (the tough cellulose outer shell has been opened to improve bioavailability and binding capacity).

The broken cell wall format matters because it:

- Increases surface area for binding
- Improves digestibility
- Enhances nutrient absorption

What Broken Cell Wall Chlorella Provides

1. Binding Capacity – Chlorella's fibrous structure and surface properties allow it to bind certain compounds in the digestive tract, such as microbial byproducts, environmental toxins, bile-bound waste, and certain heavy metals. In the parasite detox protocol, it functions as the primary binder during antimicrobial die-off.
2. Chlorophyll – Chlorella is naturally rich in chlorophyll. Chlorophyll supports antioxidant activity, cellular protection, gentle internal deodorizing effects, and liver support during detox, which contributes to tissue resilience during active detox phases.
3. Trace Minerals – Chlorella contains naturally occurring magnesium, iron, zinc, and other trace elements. These support metabolic processes while detoxification is underway, helping prevent mineral depletion during elimination cycles.
4. Protein and Amino Acids – Chlorella contains plant-based protein and essential amino acids that support tissue repair, immune function, and general cellular maintenance. While not a primary protein source in this protocol, it contributes nutritional support.

What Medi-Chlorella-FX Does in the Parasite Detox Protocol

During ON weeks, chlorella helps bind mobilized toxins, reduce recirculation, and support smoother elimination. During OFF weeks, it continues to assist drainage, maintain bowel support, and stabilize the intestinal terrain. Proper spacing is essential, as binders should be taken 60–90 minutes away from meals, herbs, and enzymes, and adequate hydration must be maintained.

Codeage Full Spectrum Binder+

A multi-ingredient binding formula designed to support gastrointestinal detoxification through absorption, mineral exchange, and microbial metabolite binding. Unlike single-ingredient binders, this formula combines several natural binding agents to broaden surface area and functional diversity.

Active Ingredients: Activated Charcoal, Bentonite Clay, Zeolite Clinoptilolite, Humic Acid, and Fulvic Acid

Activated Charcoal
: A highly porous carbon compound that absorbs microbial byproducts, endotoxins, and digestive waste in the gut, helping reduce recirculation during detox phases.

Bentonite Clay
: A negatively charged volcanic clay that binds positively charged particles and supports stool formation.

Zeolite Clinoptilolite
: A mineral that supports ion exchange binding, particularly for certain heavy metals and charged compounds within the gut.

Humic Acid
: A soil-derived organic compound that assists with binding metabolic waste while supporting intestinal microbial balance.

Fulvic Acid
: A low molecular weight humic compound that supports mineral transport and provides mild chelating activity during detoxification.

What Codeage Binder+ Does in the Parasite Detox Protocol

During ON weeks, this formula functions as a broad-spectrum binder, helping capture microbial debris, bile-bound waste, and endotoxins released during antimicrobial pressure. The combination approach widens coverage beyond a single binding mechanism.
During OFF weeks, it supports continued drainage, bowel regularity, and stabilization of the intestinal terrain.

As with all binders, proper timing is essential. It should be taken 60–90 minutes away from meals, supplements, herbs, and medications. Adequate hydration is required to support movement through the digestive tract and effective elimination.

Premier Aloe

Premier Aloe is a whole-leaf aloe vera supplement designed to support digestive integrity, soothe irritation, and promote balanced elimination during detoxification cycles.

Active Ingredient: Organic Aloe Vera (whole leaf) *(Aloe barbadensis)* Containing min. 11% acemannan – Premier Aloe uses carefully processed aloe vera to preserve its naturally occurring polysaccharides and soothing compounds while removing excessive anthraquinones that can irritate the bowel when overused. Whole-leaf aloe provides a broader spectrum of supportive plant compounds compared to isolated extracts.

What Aloe Provides

1. Mucosal Soothing Support – Aloe contains polysaccharides which helps soothe intestinal lining, supports mucosal integrity, calms irritation during antimicrobial die-off, and reduces gut sensitivity. During detox, the intestinal lining can become reactive. Aloe helps maintain barrier stability.
2. Gentle Motility Support – Aloe supports normal bowel movement without harsh stimulation. It helps encourage smooth elimination and also can reduce mild constipation. This is important during antimicrobial protocols where stagnation increases recirculation.
3. Anti-Inflammatory Support – Aloe contains naturally occurring plant compounds that help moderate inflammatory signaling in the digestive tract. This is particularly helpful for bloating, mild cramping, and irritation during detox transitions. It pairs well with turmeric for broader inflammatory modulation.
4. Gut Barrier Support – Aloe supports the structural integrity of the gut lining. During antimicrobial cycling, maintaining barrier integrity reduces leaky gut stress, food reactivity, and immune overactivation. It functions as a stabilizer during microbial shifts.

What Premier Aloe Does in the Parasite Detox Protocol

During ON weeks, aloe soothes the gut lining during die-off, supports bowel regularity, and helps protect mucosal tissue. During OFF weeks, it continues to assist tissue repair, supports the restoration phase, and maintains elimination without stimulation. Best taken with dinner to support overnight repair, aloe helps balance the intensity of antimicrobial herbs, supports elimination without dependency, protects intestinal tissue, and integrates well with bile support and binders.

Premier Turmeric

Premier Turmeric is a concentrated turmeric formula designed to support healthy inflammatory balance, liver function, and tissue protection during detoxification cycles.

Active Ingredients:

Organic Turmeric (rhizome) *(Curcuma longa)*
Turmeric root contains naturally occurring curcuminoids and volatile oils that support healthy inflammatory signaling and antioxidant protection. Whole-root turmeric provides a broader phytochemical profile beyond isolated curcumin alone.

Turmeric Extract (standardized curcuminoids)
Standardized extract increases the concentration of curcuminoids — the compounds most associated with turmeric's anti-inflammatory and antioxidant properties. This enhances potency while maintaining whole-root synergy.

What Turmeric Provides

1. Inflammatory Modulation – During antimicrobial protocols, microbial die-off can increase inflammatory signaling. Turmeric helps support balanced cytokine response, reduce discomfort during detox, calm systemic inflammatory flare, and support joint and muscle comfort. This becomes especially important in Phases 2 and 3.
2. Liver Support – Turmeric supports Phase I and Phase II liver detox pathways, antioxidant protection within liver tissue, and healthy bile production. It works synergistically with BiliVen to promote efficient toxin processing.
3. Antioxidant Protection – Detoxification increases oxidative stress. Turmeric provides antioxidant compounds that help protect cellular membranes, support mitochondrial stability, reduce oxidative burden during toxin mobilization. This helps prevent fatigue and inflammatory overload.
4. Gut Integrity Support – Turmeric contributes to maintenance of gut barrier integrity, reduction of intestinal irritation, and support of mucosal healing. It pairs well with aloe for digestive protection.

What Premier Turmeric Does in the Parasite Detox Protocol

During ON weeks, turmeric helps moderate the inflammatory response associated with die-off, supports liver processing of toxins, and enhances bile flow. During OFF weeks, it continues to protect hepatic tissue and supports recovery and recalibration of the liver. It is best taken at bedtime to encourage overnight repair.

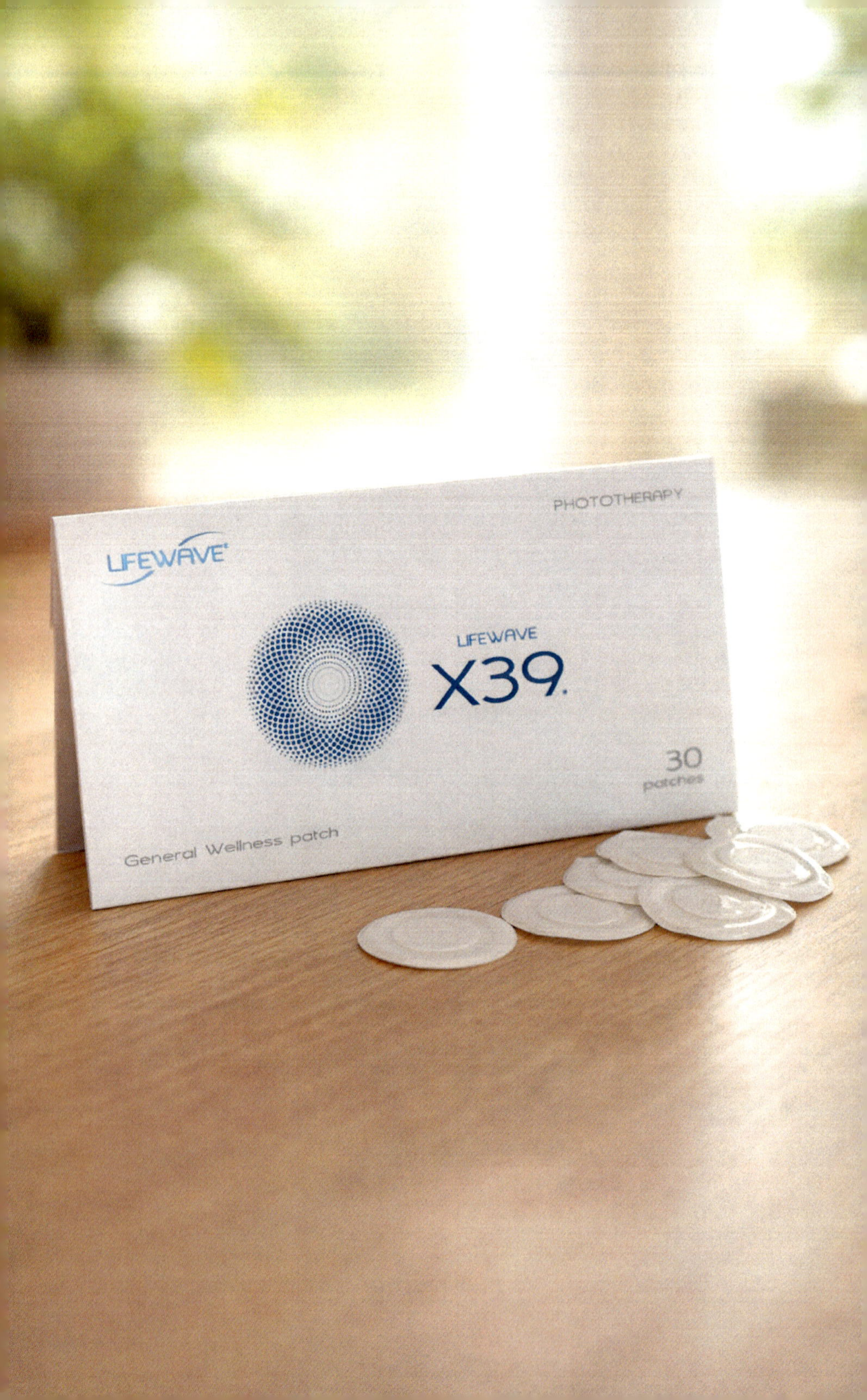
PHOTOTHERAPY
LIFEWAVE
LIFEWAVE
X39.
30
patches
General Wellness patch

CHAPTER 12
PEPTIDE SUPPORT PATCHES

SHOPPING LIST:
From LifeWave www.LifeWave.com/vitality

- 3 sleeves LifeWave® X39® patches
- 2 sleeves LifeWave® Glutathione patches
- 2 sleeves LifeWave® Aeon® patches

PHOTOTHERAPY PATCHES
Some people move through a parasite protocol smoothly. Others feel the strain more quickly. The difference often comes down to how well the body regulates stress chemistry, oxidative burden, detox capacity, and repair signaling while clearing debris.

Parasite cleansing is about eliminating organisms *and* managing the physiologic ripple effects that follow immune activation, tissue irritation, and metabolic clearance. When regulatory systems are strong, the process feels steadier. When they are taxed, symptoms can intensify.

In addition to foundational support such as hydration, minerals, binders, bowel regularity, and liver support, it is wise to incorporate specific phototherapy peptide patches designed to stimulate the body's own regulatory pathways rather than introduce exogenous compounds.

Three important patches with published research are LifeWave® X39®, Glutathione, and Aeon. You may find the links to the research on www.PatchEDU.com. Each supports a different aspect of physiologic regulation through peptide increase as follows:

- X39® supports endogenous GHK-Cu and repair signaling
- Glutathione supports antioxidant and detox pathways
- Aeon® supports stress modulation and autonomic balance

It is important to note that LifeWave® patches are not anti-parasitic agents. They are supportive regulators that help the body maintain resilience during preparation and active clearing phases of a parasite detox.

X39 PATCHES AND GHK-CU

Some support tools stimulate what the body already produces instead of adding to it in the way herbal supplements do. One example is the use of the LifeWave® X39® patch, which has been studied for its ability to elevate endogenous GHK-Cu. This is a very important copper-binding peptide that functions as a powerful regulator of inflammation, repair, and tissue resilience.

Proven Effect: Increased Endogenous GHK-Cu

In a double-blind, randomized controlled human study, adults aged 40–80 wore the X39® patch or a control patch for one week. At the end of the study, subjects using X39® showed a statistically significant rise in circulating GHK-Cu levels compared with controls. This means the body itself produced more GHK-Cu while using the patch — not as a supplement, not as an external compound, but internally elevated through physiological signaling.

This is important because GHK-Cu isn't an "add-on nutrient." It is an endogenous signaling molecule, like a master communicator that helps coordinate multiple tissue-level processes.

It is also important to recognize that natural GHK-Cu levels decline with age. Research has shown that circulating GHK-Cu concentrations are significantly higher in young adults and progressively decrease over time. Because many individuals beginning parasite cleansing protocols are over 40, supporting endogenous GHK-Cu may help restore signaling capacity that has gradually diminished. Using the X39® patch can help re-establish balanced regulatory communication that supports inflammation resolution, tissue repair, and antioxidant resilience.

What GHK-Cu Does in the Body

1. Modulates Inflammation – During a parasite cleanse, the immune system activates, inflammatory cytokines rise, stress pathways kick in, and the body mobilizes macrophages and other immune cells to deal with debris. GHK-Cu does not blunt this response; instead, it helps the body regulate it.

   Scientific studies show that GHK-Cu can:

   - Reduce expression of pro-inflammatory genes
   - Decrease key inflammatory mediators such as TNF-a and IL-6
   - Improve balance between inflammatory signaling and resolution pathways

This reflects greater regulation rather than complete suppression, allowing for controlled inflammatory signaling that remains effective. Inflammation is not the enemy; it is the body's protective response and a critical signal for immune function. The goal is not to eliminate inflammation altogether, but to support a properly regulated response that clears efficiently without excessive tissue stress. In parasite protocols, this can translate into less symptom flare while maintaining effective clearance.

2. Supports Tissue Repair and Remodeling – Parasite cleansing can cause cellular stress, mild mucosal irritation, and an increase in oxidative by-products. GHK-Cu supports the body's repair systems by stimulating fibroblast migration, increasing collagen synthesis, promoting angiogenesis (healthy microcirculation), and activating genes linked to wound repair. These roles are well documented in the scientific literature, where GHK-Cu has been shown to accelerate recovery in models of tissue injury and oxidative stress.
3. Enhances Antioxidant Signaling – Parasite die-off is often misunderstood as "toxicity." In reality, it is an oxidative burst. This is when immune cells produce free radicals to help neutralize antigens and debris. If antioxidant pathways lag, symptoms can intensify. GHK-Cu helps shift the balance toward resiliency by increasing expression of antioxidant enzymes, supporting glutathione-related pathways, and reducing oxidative stress markers at the gene expression level. This aligns with a smoother detox experience by balancing oxidation more effectively.

Why Increased GHK-Cu Matters in the Parasite Detox

- Parasite elimination involves tissue interaction, immune activation, oxidative burst activity, and increased demand for repair signaling. When the body has more GHK-Cu available, inflammation becomes more regulated, repair mechanisms are more efficient, and the antioxidant response is stronger.
- In practical terms for someone in a parasite protocol, this can show up as less pronounced die-off symptoms, faster recovery of irritated tissues, more stable energy and mood, better oxidative balance, and greater resilience through stress signaling cycles.
- GHK-Cu does not kill parasites directly, and it does not replace foundational protocol work (bowel regularity, minerals, binders, liver support, hydration, etc.). Instead, it supports the body's own regulatory architecture, which is the very system that determines whether a cleanse feels like chaos or controlled progress.

AEON PATCHES AND STRESS ADAPTATION

Parasite protocols place measurable demands on the autonomic nervous system. Stress signaling can influence bile flow, gut motility, immune activation, and inflammatory tone. Supporting adaptive nervous system balance can therefore improve how the body tolerates active clearing. The LifeWave® Aeon® patch has been studied for its influence on autonomic balance, amino-acid related pathways, and markers associated with adaptive nervous system function.

Proven Effects: Autonomic Balance & Neurochemical Regulation

Studies examining the Aeon® patch show measurable changes in markers tied to the body's stress and regulatory systems. In a randomized placebo-controlled pilot trial, participants using Aeon® exhibited statistically significant changes in levels of selected amino acids including glutamate, L-DOPA, cysteine, glutamine, serine, and proline, within 24 hours compared with placebo. These changes suggest shifts in biochemical pathways linked to neurotransmitter balance, antioxidant pathways, and stress adaptation. Additionally, heart rate variability (HRV) testing associated Aeon® use with a shift toward increased parasympathetic activity, indicating a calmer, more balanced autonomic state.

These findings do not imply that Aeon® directly creates neurotransmitters in isolation, but rather that Aeon® patch use appears to correlate with measurable changes in markers that are linked to adaptive regulation and stress response pathways.

What This Means in the Body

1. Supports Parasympathetic Dominance

   The autonomic nervous system has two major arms:

   - The sympathetic ("fight, flight, defend")
   - The parasympathetic ("rest, digest, regulate")

   During detoxification and immune activation, when you are undergoing a parasite detox, sympathetic dominance can escalate:

   - Nervous tension
   - Digestive slowdown
   - Hormonal swings
   - Energy fluctuations

   In contrast, parasympathetic activity supports:

   - Smoother digestion
   - Improved elimination
   - Balanced mood
   - More stable energy rhythms

Data from HRV testing shows Aeon® use correlates with a shift toward parasympathetic balance. This means a more regulated, calmer physiologic state that helps coordinate immune and metabolic clearance without excessive stress activation.

2. Supports Biochemical Adaptation
   The pilot clinical data showing changes in key amino acids and related metabolites suggests Aeon patch use correlates with shifts in pathways that intersect with:
   - Glutamate – excitatory signaling and precursor to GABA
   - L-DOPA – motivation and dopaminergic pathways
   - Cysteine – a precursor for antioxidants including glutathione
   - Glutamine – important for immune cell fuel
   - Serine & Proline – stress modulation and tissue support

   In a parasite cleanse, adaptive stress response is often just as important as microbial clearance. A regulated nervous system supports digestive motility, immune coordination, liver function, and emotional equilibrium, all of which contribute to smoother protocol progress.

Why Aeon Matters in the Parasite Detox
Much of the discomfort people associate with cleansing comes from more than pathogen exposure alone. It often arises from:

- Nervous system hyperactivation
- Stress hormone dysregulation
- Miscommunication between organ systems
- Overstimulation of immune pathways

The Aeon patch supports adaptive regulation by helping the body shift toward physiological balance where stress responses are appropriate rather than excessive.

In practical terms, this can translate into:

- Improved digestive ease during clearing phases
- More regulated mood and energy
- Smoother sleep patterns
- Less reactive stress signaling

This support layer aligns with the cleansing process, allowing foundational mechanisms (bowel regularity, liver support, binder timing, hydration, antioxidant pathways) to function in a calmer biochemical environment.

GLUTATHIONE PATCH AND DETOX PATHWAYS

Some supportive tools work by enhancing the body's own biochemical capacity rather than introducing exogenous compounds. The LifeWave Glutathione patch is one such tool, studied for its ability to influence the body's own glutathione status. Glutathione is a cornerstone molecule in cellular antioxidant defense and phase II detoxification pathways.

Glutathione homeostasis is dynamic and demand-dependent. Levels decline during periods of immune activation, xenobiotic exposure, and increased oxidative stress due to accelerated utilization. During a parasite cleanse, glutathione demand rises as the body processes endotoxins, inflammatory mediators, and mobilized environmental compounds. If synthesis and recycling are insufficient to meet this increased demand, redox imbalance may develop. Supporting endogenous glutathione production during this phase helps maintain oxidative equilibrium and reduces the risk of depletion becoming a limiting factor in tissue recovery and detoxification efficiency.

Proven Effects – Increased Endogenous Glutathione

In a human clinical pilot study, participants wearing the LifeWave Glutathione patch showed a statistically significant increase in circulating glutathione levels compared with controls. Urinary mercury levels also increased in some participants, suggesting mobilization of metals, although the exact mechanism and causation remain areas for further research. Importantly, the study measured endogenous glutathione, meaning the body's own glutathione levels were elevated in response to patch use rather than being supplied from an external source. This distinction is key: the patch is not a glutathione supplement. It is a bioregulatory stimulus that supports internal glutathione production and balance.

What Glutathione Does in the Body

1. Central Antioxidant Defense

   Glutathione is often called the body's "master antioxidant."

   It directly participates in:

   - Neutralizing reactive oxygen species (ROS)
   - Regenerating other antioxidants (e.g., vitamins C and E)
   - Supporting redox balance at the cellular level

   During a parasite cleanse, immune activation increases ROS production. Without sufficient antioxidant capacity, oxidative stress can build, which may show up as headaches, fatigue, or irritability. Supporting glutathione helps the body manage oxidative burden without hindering the immune response.

2. Phase II Detoxification Support
   The liver's phase II detox pathways rely heavily on glutathione conjugation. This is the process by which toxins, metabolites, and cellular debris are bound and prepared for excretion. Glutathione participates in conjugation of lipophilic compounds, enhancement of bile flow and toxin transport, and support for glutathione S-transferase (GST) enzyme activity. Elevated glutathione status supports these pathways, helping the body move by-products of clearing out more efficiently.
3. Heavy Metal Mobilization Signaling
   In the clinical pilot study, some participants exhibited increased urinary mercury. While the study concluded that a direct mechanistic link was not definitively established, the observation is consistent with glutathione's known biochemical role: glutathione is involved in binding and transporting heavy metals as part of detoxification metabolism. In parasite protocols, mobilizing metals and other stored compounds can be part of the clearance phase. Supporting endogenous glutathione may help the body handle mobilized metals more effectively by assisting in sequestration and excretion pathways.

Why Glutathione Matters in the Parasite Detox

Parasite die-off and immune activation supports:

- Oxidative stress from immune responses
- Metabolite and endotoxin mobilization
- Phase II liver detoxification demand
- Cellular redox balance challenge

When glutathione is supported and elevated:

- Cellular antioxidant protection increases
- Phase II detox pathways function more efficiently
- Oxidative stress is more evenly regulated
- Metabolic waste handling is improved

This does not mean inflammation is shut down or immune function is suppressed. Glutathione enhances regulatory capacity by allowing the body to process oxidative and metabolic load more effectively while the immune system does its job.

You can think of glutathione as the body's internal fire control system. The immune response may light a controlled burn to clear debris, but without regulation, that burn can spread and damage surrounding tissue. Glutathione does not extinguish the fire. It contains it, directs it, and ensures that once the necessary work is complete, restoration can begin.

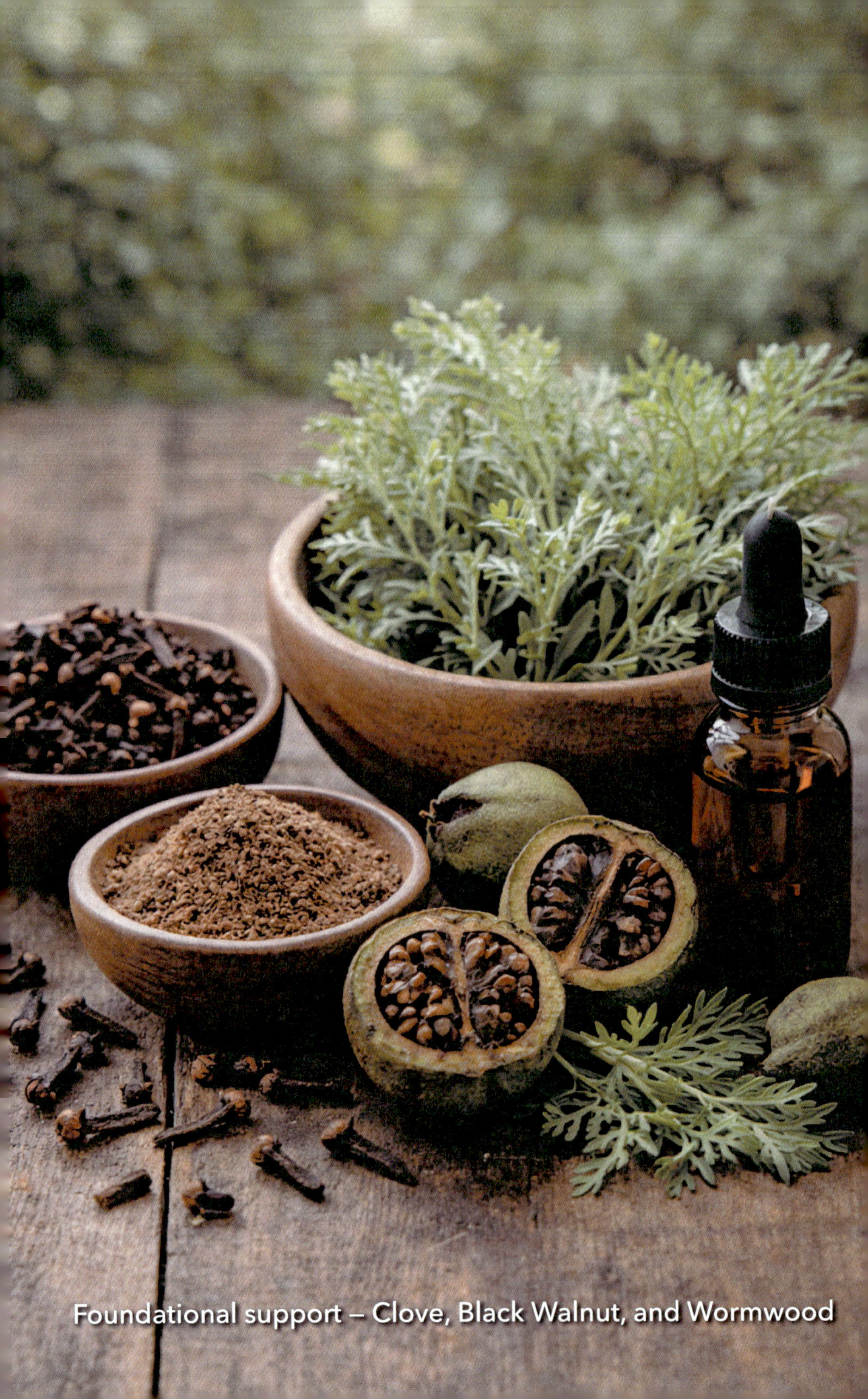

Foundational support – Clove, Black Walnut, and Wormwood

CHAPTER 13
THE PROTOCOL

Every effective protocol follows a pattern. It is not random, not rushed, and not reactive, but well-structured. Parasites are adaptive organisms. They respond to pressure. If pressure is constant and unrelenting, they can shift survival strategies. If pressure is too aggressive too quickly, the host often suffers more than the organism. A thoughtful protocol respects both biology and timing.

This section outlines a ten-week structured progression designed to prepare the terrain, apply targeted antimicrobial support, allow strategic rest, and then consolidate restoration. The rhythm matters. Escalation matters. Recovery windows matter. You will notice that this protocol is not a straight line, but rather, it moves in cycles.

PROTOCOL PATTERN

Week 1 – Preparation
Week 2 – Phase 1 (active detox)
Week 3 – Phase 1 (active detox)
Week 4 – Phase 2 (rest)
Week 5 – Phase 3 (escalation detox)
Week 6 – Phase 3 (escalation detox)
Week 7 – Phase 2 (rest)
Week 8 – Phase 1 (active detox)
Week 9 – Phase 1 (active detox)
Week 10 – Restoration

The preparation week builds drainage capacity and stabilizes digestion before antimicrobial pressure begins. Phase 1 introduces targeted herbal support in a measured way. Phase 2 intentionally reduces antimicrobial load to allow immune recalibration and microbial stabilization. Phase 3 increases intensity for deeper reduction. Restoration consolidates gains, rebuilds the microbiome, and supports long-term equilibrium.

This wave-like structure reduces overwhelm, supports bile flow and bowel function, protects beneficial flora, and minimizes unnecessary inflammatory flare. It also acknowledges something important: the body does not heal under constant assault. It heals when challenge and recovery are balanced.

Move through each week steadily and don't rush escalation or skip rest. Observe your responses carefully and hydrate well.

PREPARATION – Week 1

Before antimicrobial pressure begins, the body must be ready. Preparation week is about opening drainage pathways, stabilizing digestion, supporting bile flow, and ensuring consistent elimination. When the liver, bile, bowel, and microbiome are functioning well, the system can handle microbial reduction with far less discomfort. This phase builds resilience first so that when pressure increases, the body responds efficiently rather than reactively.

DAILY STRUCTURE

<u>Morning – Upon Waking</u>
(Before breakfast on empty stomach, 30–45 minutes before food.)
- 8 ounces warm water with the juice of ½ fresh lemon
- 3 capsules Medi-Chlorella-FX or 1 capsule Codeage Binder+

<u>Patches</u>
- 12 hours on during waking hours
- LifeWave X39, Aeon, and Glutathione patches
- LifeWave X39/Aeon worn daily; Glutathione worn every other day

<u>Breakfast</u>
Protein-forward meal with healthy fats included (see *Ketovore24* book*)
- 2 capsules BiliVen
- 1 capsule Microbiome-18
- 1 serving digestive enzyme complex such as Premier Digest

<u>One Hour Before Lunch</u>
(At least 60–90 minutes away from food and supplements.)
- 3 capsules Medi-Chlorella-FX or 1 capsule Codeage Binder+
- Hydrate – binders require water to move efficiently through the bowel

<u>Dinner</u>
Lower carbohydrate and anti-inflammatory meal (see *Ketovore24* book*)
- 2 capsules BiliVen
- 1 capsule Microbiome-18
- 2 capsules Premier Aloe or Global Healing Aloe Vera

<u>Before Bed</u>
(On an empty stomach, at least 2 hours after dinner.)
- 1–2 capsules Premier Turmeric
- 1 serving Magnesium glycinate or Premier Calcium Magnesium Plus

* The *Ketovore24* book is available at www.PatchEDU.com

PHASE 1 (ACTIVE DETOX) – Weeks 2 and 3

This is the gentle entry phase. We introduce antimicrobial pressure slowly to protect bile flow, bind intentionally to support proper elimination, and monitor closely so adjustments can be made as needed.

DAILY STRUCTURE

<u>Morning – Upon Waking</u>
(Before breakfast on empty stomach, 30–45 minutes before food.)
- Hydrate with a glass of pure water
- 1 capsule ParaStat
- 1 capsule Paratosin
- 1 capsule Gaia Microbiome Cleanse

NOTE: Taking antimicrobials away from food allows for more direct contact and reduces interference with absorption.

<u>Patches</u>
- 12 hours on during waking hours
- LifeWave X39, Aeon, and Glutathione patches
- LifeWave X39/Aeon worn daily; Glutathione worn every other day

<u>Breakfast</u>
Protein-forward meal with healthy fats included (see *Ketovore24* book*)
- 2 capsules BiliVen
- 1 capsule Microbiome-18

NOTE: Bile support remains essential as microbial debris increases.

<u>One Hour Before Lunch</u>
(At least 60–90 minutes away from food and supplements.)
- 3 capsules Medi-Chlorella-FX or 1 capsule Codeage Binder+
- Hydrate – binders require water to move efficiently through the bowel

<u>Dinner</u>
Lower carbohydrate and anti-inflammatory meal (see *Ketovore24* book*)
- 2 capsules BiliVen
- 2 capsules Premier Aloe or Global Healing Aloe Vera

<u>Before Bed</u>
(On an empty stomach, at least 2 hours after dinner.)
- 1 capsule Gaia Microbiome Cleanse
- 1 capsule ParaStat
- 1 capsule Paratosin
- 1–2 capsules Premier Turmeric

* The *Ketovore24* book is available at www.PatchEDU.com

PHASE 2 (REST & RESTORATION) – Week 4

This is the intentional pause. Phase 2 lasts one week only and serves as the reset between active antimicrobial cycles. We temporarily remove parasite-specific formulas while continuing foundational support, liver flow, binding, and cellular repair. This week is not passive. It is strategic. We allow the body to recalibrate, strengthen the terrain, and rebuild microbial balance before entering the next active phase.

What Changes in Phase 2

- ParaStat is paused
- Paratosin is paused
- Microbiome-18 is increased
- Premier Probiotic may be added (optional)
- All other foundational supplements and patches continue

DAILY STRUCTURE

Morning – Upon Waking
(Before breakfast on empty stomach, 30–45 minutes before food.)

- Hydrate with a full glass of pure water
- No parasite formulas during this week

Patches

- 12 hours on during waking hours
- LifeWave X39, Aeon, and Glutathione patches
- LifeWave X39/Aeon worn daily; Glutathione worn every other day

Breakfast
Protein-forward meal with healthy fats included (see *Ketovore24* book*)

- 2 capsules BiliVen
- 2 capsules Microbiome-18
  NOTE: Microbiome-18 is intentionally increased during this week to reinforce microbial balance.

One Hour Before Lunch
(At least 60–90 minutes away from food and supplements.)

- 3 capsules Medi-Chlorella-FX or 1 capsule Codeage Binder+
- Hydrate well

NOTE: Binding continues during the restoration week. The body is still clearing residual debris from Phase 1. Keeping elimination pathways open prevents recirculation. If detox symptoms have resolved and stools are consistent, chlorella may be reduced slightly. If symptoms linger, maintain the full dose.

* The *Ketovore24* book is available at www.PatchEDU.com

Dinner
Lower carbohydrate and anti-inflammatory meal (see *Ketovore24* book*)

- 2 capsules BiliVen
- 2 capsules Microbiome-18
- 2 capsules Premier Aloe or Global Healing Aloe Vera
  NOTE: Aloe continues to support mucosal integrity and bowel motility. Microbiome-18 remains elevated to strengthen gut resilience before returning to active antimicrobial pressure.

Before Bed
(On an empty stomach, at least 2 hours after dinner.)

- 1–2 capsules Premier Turmeric
  NOTE: Turmeric supports inflammatory balance and liver function.
- 1 capsule Premier Probiotic
  NOTE: Bedtime is often ideal for probiotics. Gastric activity is lower, antimicrobial formulas are paused, and beneficial organisms have a greater opportunity to colonize.

Why the One-Week Pause Matters
Continuous antimicrobial pressure without rest can disrupt beneficial flora and increase inflammatory load. A structured one-week restoration phase allows:

- Microbial recalibration
- Gut lining repair
- Bile rhythm stabilization
- Nervous system recovery

Many individuals report improved energy, steadier digestion, reduced bloating, more consistent bowel patterns, deeper sleep, stabilized mood, and clearer thinking during the restoration week. Inflammatory flares often settle. These changes reflect decreased antigen load and reduced endotoxin circulation. When antimicrobial pressure pauses, the immune system recalibrates, cytokine signaling settles, bile flow normalizes, the gut lining repairs, and microbial communities rebalance rather than react.

Feeling better does not mean the work is finished or that intensity has been lost. This week is a physiological integration window. Consolidation prevents overactivation, reduces resistance risk, protects beneficial flora, and strengthens the terrain for the next escalation phase while honoring the body's adaptive rhythms.

Think of it like strength training. Muscle does not grow during the lift. It grows during recovery. Phase 2 reinforces the foundation before you embark on a deeper cleanse in Phase 3.

* The *Ketovore24* book is available at www.PatchEDU.com

PHASE 3 (ESCALATION DETOX) – Weeks 5 and 6

This is where we deepen the work. Your terrain has been supported. Your microbiome has been strengthened. Bile flow has been protected. Now we reintroduce antimicrobial pressure at a higher therapeutic level.

Phase 3 increases dosing intentionally. This is not aggressive for the sake of aggression. It is strategic escalation after preparation. Listen closely to your body during this phase. Escalation works best when elimination pathways remain open and hydration is strong.

What Changes in Phase 3

- ParaStat increases to 2 capsules twice daily
- Paratosin increases to 2 capsules twice daily
- Microbiome-18 returns to maintenance level
- Optional Premier Probiotic may continue if well tolerated
- Foundational supports and patches remain in place

DAILY STRUCTURE

<u>Morning</u>
(Before breakfast on empty stomach, 30–45 minutes before food.)

- 1 capsule Gaia Microbiome Cleanse
- 2 capsules ParaStat
- 2 capsules Paratosin
- Hydrate with a full glass of pure water

NOTE: Escalation works best when taken on a truly empty stomach.

<u>Patches</u>

- 12 hours on during waking hours
- LifeWave X39 and Aeon worn daily
- LifeWave Glutathione worn every other day

NOTE: As antimicrobial pressure increases, cellular repair and glutathione support remain essential.

<u>Breakfast</u>
Protein-forward meal with healthy fats included (see *Ketovore24* book*)

- 2 capsules BiliVen
- 1 capsule Microbiome-18
- Optional – 1 capsule Premier Probiotic

NOTE: Microbiome-18 returns to maintenance dosing during active escalation. We maintain terrain support without competing heavily with antimicrobial action.

* The *Ketovore24* book is available at www.PatchEDU.com

<u>One Hour Before Lunch</u>
(At least 60–90 minutes away from food and supplements.)

- 3 capsules Medi-Chlorella-FX or 1 capsule Codeage Binder+
- Hydrate well

NOTE: If detox symptoms increase during escalation, binders may be increased slightly for a few days. Binders prevent recirculation of toxins/die-off and reduce inflammatory flares.

<u>Dinner</u>
Lower carbohydrate and anti-inflammatory meal (see *Ketovore24* book*)

- 1 dropper (30 drops) Gaia Wormwood Black Walnut Supreme
- 2 capsules BiliVen
- 2 capsules Premier Aloe or Global Healing Aloe Vera

NOTE: Fiber balance, bowel motility, and bile rhythm must remain strong in this phase. Constipation will amplify symptoms.

<u>Before Bed</u>
(On an empty stomach, at least 2 hours after dinner.)

- 1 capsule Gaia Microbiome Cleanse
- 2 capsules ParaStat
- 2 capsules Paratosin
- 1–2 capsules Premier Turmeric

NOTE: Some individuals may prefer taking the evening antimicrobial dose 1–2 hours after dinner rather than immediately before bed if stomach sensitivity occurs.

What to Expect During Phase 3 Escalation
Because dosing increases, some people may experience temporary fatigue, mild headaches, changes in stool, skin flares, and/or sleep shifts. These are signals to adjust support, not abandon the protocol. Increase hydration. Ensure daily bowel movements. Consider increasing binders briefly if symptoms rise. If symptoms feel excessive or prolonged, reduce antimicrobial dosing back to Phase 1 levels for several days before attempting escalation again.

Why Escalation Is Structured
A structured escalation is essential because parasites adapt, their biofilms provide protective shielding, and dormant organisms can resurface. Increasing the therapeutic window after adequate preparation improves the likelihood of a meaningful reduction in parasite burden. Maintain hydration and remain attentive to your body's signals.

After completing Phase 3, go to Phase 2 (rest), then Phase 1 (active detox), and finish on Week 10 with the Restoration Phase.

* The *Ketovore24* book is available at www.PatchEDU.com

RESTORATION – Week 10

Week 10 follows the exact structure of Phase 2 (Rest and Restoration) with a few slight adjustments as seen below. All parasite-specific formulas remain paused, and foundational support continues as written in Phase 2. The difference in this final week is intention and tapering. We are no longer preparing for another antimicrobial cycle. We are stabilizing and securing the gains of the protocol. BiliVen, aloe, turmeric, hydration, and patch support continue exactly as outlined in Phase 2.

Add the Following in Week 10:

- Maintain the increased Microbiome-18 dosing for the entire week
- Continue nightly probiotic support
- Taper binder use during the second half of the week if bowel movements are consistent and detox symptoms have resolved
- Add trace minerals and collagen to reinforce nutrient repletion

Why Week 10 Matters

This week consolidates your progress. Your microbial balance gets anchored, the gut lining continues repair, bile rhythm stabilizes, and your immune signaling settles into regulatory balance. Phase 2 resets the terrain before escalation. The Restoration Week 10 secures the terrain before maintenance.

What to Expect After Completion

Most individuals notice steadier digestion, improved bowel rhythm, clearer thinking, and more consistent energy by the end of Week 10. Some may continue to see gradual improvement over the next several weeks as the microbiome stabilizes and detox pathways normalize.
It is appropriate to remain observant during the month following completion. Monitor bowel consistency, sleep quality, skin changes, and overall resilience. Subtle improvements often continue as your body terrain settles.

When to Consider Another Cycle

A repeat cycle is commonly performed once per year as part of routine terrain maintenance. This annual rhythm supports microbial recalibration and digestive resilience, particularly in modern environments where exposure through food, travel, water, and animals is common.

For individuals with higher exposure risk, frequent travel, agricultural or animal contact, chronic digestive vulnerability, or a previously significant burden, a structured cycle every six months may be appropriate. Semi-annual maintenance can provide a steadier rhythm for those who tend to experience recurrent symptoms.

If symptoms gradually re-emerge, such as bloating, irregular bowel patterns, unexplained fatigue, skin flares, increased food sensitivities, or sleep disturbance, reassessment after an 8–12 week rest interval is reasonable. The body benefits from a period of stabilization before reintroducing antimicrobial pressure. This interval allows microbial communities, immune signaling, and detoxification pathways to recalibrate fully before another structured intervention.

Not everyone requires frequent cycles. Some individuals maintain long-term stability through consistent nutrition, hydration, mineral sufficiency, bowel regularity, and periodic microbiome support without repeating the full protocol for many months. The appropriate frequency should reflect exposure patterns, symptom recurrence, and overall resilience rather than routine alone.

Structured intervention works best when it is cyclical and intentional. For many, annual maintenance is sufficient. For others with higher exposure or persistent terrain instability, a semi-annual (every six months) rhythm may be more supportive.

Maintenance Principles

- Prioritize protein-forward, anti-inflammatory meals
- Limit or eliminate sugars and processed carbohydrates
- Maintain hydration and mineral balance
- Support regular bowel movements
- Use binders situationally
- Continue microbiome support as needed

Closing Guidance

Completion of the parasite detox protocol marks a return to steady-state physiology. The structured phases have applied controlled antimicrobial pressure, supported elimination, and reinforced repair. Week 10 consolidates that work. From here, the focus shifts to maintenance. Continue prioritizing digestive rhythm, hydration, mineral sufficiency, and nutrient-dense meals. Allow the system to function without additional intervention unless symptoms clearly indicate otherwise.

There is no advantage in extending antimicrobial intensity beyond the defined window. Periodic, structured cycles are more supportive than continuous pressure. The goal of this protocol was a recalibration of terrain, restoration of balance, and strengthening of resilience. With that foundation in place, the body is equipped to maintain stability moving forward.

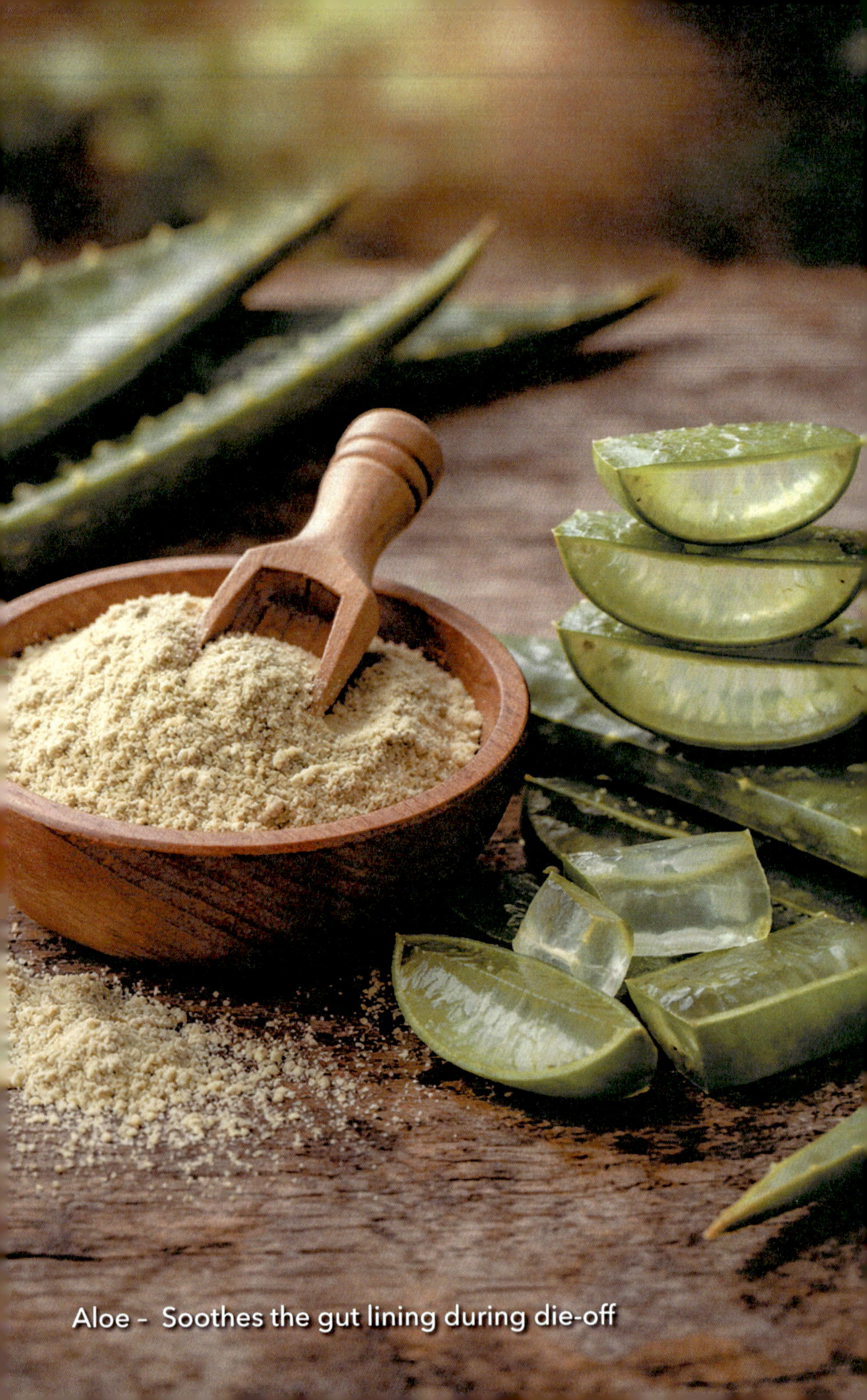

Aloe – Soothes the gut lining during die-off

CHAPTER 14
TROUBLESHOOTING

This appendix is designed to help you assess, adjust, and proceed with clarity. Parasite cleansing requires observation and adjustments.

COMMON RESPONSES & WHAT TO DO

Headache, Brain Fog, Irritability
Often related to endotoxin circulation or sluggish elimination.
Consider:
- Increase hydration
- Add or increase binder support
- Support bile flow (BiliVen, bitters, healthy fats)
- Ensure daily bowel movement

NOTE: If symptoms persist, reduce antimicrobial pressure temporarily.

Constipation
Detox pathways must remain open.
Consider:
- Increase water intake
- Add magnesium if appropriate
- Increase aloe or fiber support
- Gentle movement or walking daily

NOTE: Do not escalate antimicrobials if bowels are not regular.

Loose Stools
Can indicate excessive antimicrobial pressure or gut irritation.
Consider:
- Reduce dosing temporarily
- Add microbiome support
- Ensure meals contain adequate protein and healthy fats
- Evaluate stress and sleep

NOTE: Stability precedes escalation.

Skin Flare-Ups or Rashes
Often linked to toxin mobilization.
Consider:
- Increase binders
- Support liver and bile flow
- Confirm adequate hydration
- Avoid introducing new supplements during flare

NOTE: Monitor symptoms. If rash is severe or accompanied by systemic symptoms, seek medical evaluation.

Fatigue
May reflect immune response, detox, or inadequate nourishment.
Consider:
- Increase protein intake
- Evaluate mineral status
- Ensure adequate sleep
- Consider extending a restoration week

NOTE: Energy should gradually improve over time.

WHEN TO PAUSE

Pause antimicrobial agents if:
- No bowel movement for 48 hours
- Severe abdominal pain
- Persistent vomiting
- Signs of allergic reaction
- Significant dizziness or fainting

NOTE: Stabilize first, then resume when elimination and hydration are steady.

WHEN TO EXTEND A PHASE

Extend a phase if:
- Symptoms spike with escalation
- Bowel function becomes irregular
- Sleep becomes significantly disrupted
- Inflammatory symptoms increase

NOTE: Lengthening a phase supports adaptation and reduces unnecessary stress on the body.

RED FLAG CHECKLIST

Seek medical care if you experience:
- High or persistent fever
- Severe abdominal pain
- Blood in stool
- Unexplained rapid weight loss
- Signs of obstruction
- New neurological symptoms

QUICK DAILY READINESS CHECK

Before increasing dosing, ask:

- Am I hydrated?
- Am I eliminating daily?
- Is my sleep stable?
- Is my inflammation trending down?
- Am I observing rather than reacting?

NOTE: If the foundation is stable, progression is appropriate.

FINAL NOTE

Parasite cleansing requires wisdom, patience, and steady observation. The body functions in systems and rhythms. When elimination pathways are open, nourishment is adequate, sleep is prioritized, and progression follows a thoughtful sequence, your terrain becomes more resilient and responsive. Sustainable change develops through consistency rather than intensity.

Every phase of this protocol is designed to respect physiology. Bile flow, bowel regularity, hydration, mineral balance, immune regulation, and microbial equilibrium all work together. Supporting these systems creates the conditions for effective reduction of microbial burden while preserving long-term stability.

Progress is often gradual. Subtle improvements in digestion, clarity, energy, and inflammatory balance signal that internal load is shifting. Maintain awareness of these markers. Adjust when necessary. Extend phases when the body requests more time. Escalate only when the foundation is stable.

Your health requires stewardship. Your role is to provide structure, nourishment, and strategic support. The body carries out the work of restoration according to the design God established within it.

Stay observant. Stay consistent. Stay steady in your sequencing. Be blessed in your journey toward greater health and wellness!

> *"Or do you not know that your body is the temple of the Holy Spirit who is in you, whom you have from God, and you are not your own? For you were bought at a price; therefore glorify God in your body and in your spirit, which are God's."* – 1 Corinthians 6:19–20 (NKJV)

BOOK REFERENCES AND SOURCES

PARASITOLOGY — FOUNDATIONAL & CLINICAL

Crompton, D. W. T., & Nesheim, M. C. (2002). Nutritional impact of intestinal helminthiasis during the human life cycle. Annual Review of Nutrition, 22, 35–59. https://doi.org/10.1146/annurev.nutr.22.120501.134539

Fletcher, S. M., Stark, D., Harkness, J., & Ellis, J. (2012). Enteric protozoa in the developed world: A public health perspective. Clinical Microbiology Reviews, 25(3), 420–449. https://doi.org/10.1128/CMR.05038-11

Hanevik, K., et al. (2009). Development of functional gastrointestinal disorders after Giardia infection. Gut, 58(7), 1092–1097. https://doi.org/10.1136/gut.2008.162644

Keiser, J., & Utzinger, J. (2008). Efficacy of current drugs against soil-transmitted helminths. JAMA, 299(16), 1937–1948. https://doi.org/10.1001/jama.299.16.1937

Stephenson, L. S., Latham, M. C., & Ottesen, E. A. (2000). Malnutrition and parasitic helminth infections. Parasitology, 121(S1), S23–S38. https://doi.org/10.1017/S0031182000006491

Torgerson, P. R., et al. (2015). World Health Organization estimates of the global burden of foodborne parasitic diseases. PLoS Medicine, 12(12), e1001920. https://doi.org/10.1371/journal.pmed.1001920

IMMUNE MODULATION & CHRONIC INFLAMMATION

Allen, J. E., & Maizels, R. M. (2011). Diversity and dialogue in immunity to helminths. Nature Reviews Immunology, 11, 375–388. https://doi.org/10.1038/nri2992

Maizels, R. M., Balic, A., Gomez-Escobar, N., Nair, M., Taylor, M. D., & Allen, J. E. (2004). Helminth parasites – masters of regulation. Immunological Reviews, 201(1), 89–116. https://doi.org/10.1111/j.0105-2896.2004.00191.x

McSorley, H. J., & Maizels, R. M. (2012). Helminth infections and host immune regulation. Clinical Microbiology Reviews, 25(4), 585–608. https://doi.org/10.1128/CMR.05040-11

GUT BARRIER, MICROBIOME & IMMUNE SIGNALING

Bischoff, S. C., et al. (2014). Intestinal permeability – a new target for disease prevention and therapy. BMC Gastroenterology, 14, 189. https://doi.org/10.1186/s12876-014-0189-7

Camilleri, M., Madsen, K., Spiller, R., Greenwood-Van Meerveld, B., & Verne, G. N. (2012). Intestinal barrier function in health and disease. Neurogastroenterology & Motility, 24(6), 503–512. https://doi.org/10.1111/j.1365-2982.2012.01921.x

Belkaid, Y., & Hand, T. W. (2014). Role of the microbiota in immunity and inflammation. Cell, 157(1), 121–141. https://doi.org/10.1016/j.cell.2014.03.011

POST-INFECTIOUS & PERSISTENT SYMPTOM RESEARCH

Hanevik, K., et al. (2014). Persisting symptoms after Giardia infection: A follow-up study. Clinical Infectious Diseases, 59(10), 1394–1400. https://doi.org/10.1093/cid/ciu629

Flegr, J. (2013). Influence of latent toxoplasmosis on human personality and behavior. Schizophrenia Bulletin, 39(1), 3–7. https://doi.org/10.1093/schbul/sbs163

GLOBALIZATION, FOOD SYSTEMS & TRANSMISSION

Robertson, L. J., Sprong, H., Ortega, Y. R., van der Giessen, J. W. B., & Fayer, R. (2014). Impacts of globalisation on foodborne parasites. Trends in Parasitology, 30(1), 37–52. https://doi.org/10.1016/j.pt.2013.09.005

Centers for Disease Control and Prevention. (2024). Giardia infection: Causes and how it spreads. https://www.cdc.gov/giardia/causes/index.html

DETOXIFICATION PHYSIOLOGY & OXIDATIVE STRESS

Lu, S. C. (2013). Glutathione synthesis. Biochimica et Biophysica Acta, 1830(5), 3143–3153. https://doi.org/10.1016/j.bbagen.2012.09.008

Pizzorno, J. (2014). Glutathione! Integrative Medicine, 13(1), 8–12. https://pmc.ncbi.nlm.nih.gov/articles/PMC4684116/

Bischoff, S. C. (2011). 'Gut health': A new objective in medicine? BMC Medicine, 9, 24. https://doi.org/10.1186/1741-7015-9-24

INFLAMMATORY RESPONSE TO PATHOGEN DIE-OFF

Author(s) not listed. (2025). Jarisch-Herxheimer reaction. In StatPearls. StatPearls Publishing. https://www.ncbi.nlm.nih.gov/books/NBK557820/

Jarczak, D., et al. (2022). Cytokine storm — definition, causes, and implications. International Journal of Molecular Sciences, 23(19), 11740. https://www.mdpi.com/1422-0067/23/19/11740

HERBAL MECHANISMS

Meshnick, S. R., Taylor, T. E., & Kamchonwongpaisan, S. (1996). Artemisinin and the antimalarial endoperoxides: From herbal remedy to targeted chemotherapy. Microbiological Reviews, 60(2), 301–315. https://doi.org/10.1128/mr.60.2.301-315.1996

Chaieb, K., Hajlaoui, H., Zmantar, T., Kahla-Nakbi, A. B., Rouabhia, M., Mahdouani, K., & Bakhrouf, A. (2007). The chemical composition and biological activity of clove essential oil, Syzygium aromaticum (L.) Merr. & L. M. Perry. Phytotherapy Research, 21(6), 501–506. https://doi.org/10.1002/ptr.2124

Khalil, R. G. (2022). Juglone as an antiparasitic, immunomodulatory, and antifibrotic agent in experimental schistosomiasis. PubMed. https://pubmed.ncbi.nlm.nih.gov/36461604/

Made in United States
North Haven, CT
05 November 2026

21766157R60058